PRAISE FOR
DEPRESSION: A WOMAN DOCTOR'S GUIDE

"This concise, no-nonsense guide is invaluable. I recognized every symptom and was grateful for the biological explanations of personality changes attributable to depression throughout the life cycle. The authors' suggestions for treatment seem just right, their optimism concerning recovery, a tonic."

—Rose Styron

"Dr. Ferber and Ms. LeVert have written an eminently readable and compassionate book that does much to explain the unique biological and psychological components of depression in women. It describes current treatments in a thoughtful and concise manner and should prompt many women to feel hope and seek help. This is a welcome addition to the literature on depression."

—Demitri F. Papolos, M.D., and Janice Papolos, authors of *Overcoming Depression*

"The book reflects three developments in the past decades: an awareness that depression is common in women; a belief that educated consumers make the best patients; and the increase in women as full partners in medicine. Ferber's book, simply stated, contains the latest information on depression applicable to both depressed men and women, but particularly sensitive to the needs of the female patient who is depressed."

—Myrna M. Weissman, Ph.D., Professor of Epidemiology in Psychiatry, College of Physicians and Surgeons of Columbia University, and Director of the Division of Clinical and Genetic Epidemiology, New York State Psychiatric Institute

BOOK YOUR PLACE ON OUR WEBSITE AND MAKE THE READING CONNECTION!

We've created a customized website just for our very special readers, where you can get the inside scoop on everything that's going on with Zebra, Pinnacle and Kensington books.

When you come online, you'll have the exciting opportunity to:

- View covers of upcoming books

- Read sample chapters

- Learn about our future publishing schedule (listed by publication month *and author*)

- Find out when your favorite authors will be visiting a city near you

- Search for and order backlist books from our online catalog

- Check out author bios and background information

- Send e-mail to your favorite authors

- Meet the Kensington staff online

- Join us in weekly chats with authors, readers and other guests

- Get writing guidelines

- AND MUCH MORE!

**Visit our website at
http://www.kensingtonbooks.com**

DEPRESSION
A
*W*OMAN
DOCTOR'S
GUIDE

**Essential Facts and
Up-to-the-Minute
Information on
Overcoming Depression**

JANE S. FERBER, M.D.

with Suzanne LeVert

KENSINGTON BOOKS
KENSINGTON PUBLISHING CORP.
hhtp://www.kensingtonbooks.com

To my family and friends, who help keep my sun shining and, with thanks, to Laurie Abkemeier, a dedicated editor and good friend.

—Suzanne LeVert

CONTENTS

DEPRESSION
A
WOMAN
DOCTOR'S GUIDE

1

▼

DEPRESSION

The Female Factor

Marilyn, a nineteen-year-old college sophomore, visits the Student Health Center complaining of fatigue so severe she's sleeping through her midterm exams. She can't concentrate and suffers frequent headaches. She attributes her problems to her recent breakup with her boyfriend, but what she doesn't admit to herself—or tell her doctor—is that she's also been bulimic off and on since her junior year in high school.

▼ Thirty-two years old and the mother of a one-year-old boy, Gail should be the picture of happiness. After all, she has everything she's always wanted: a loving husband, a healthy child, a comfortable lifestyle. Instead, she feels anxious and panicked whenever she leaves the house, virtually terrified that something will happen to her baby. She feels trapped, lonely, and guilty. She knows she isn't being a good parent to her son, but feels too paralyzed to change her situation.

▼ Beth wakes up every morning at 4:05 A.M. and cries quietly in the dark until the alarm clock rings three hours later. Even then, she lies in bed, believing that there's no point at all in getting up. At fifty-one, she looks back at her life and sees only failure, despite the fact that she's raised two children to become healthy, productive adults. This isn't a new feeling for Beth; she's been in this dark place before, but this time, with the second half of her life stretching before her, there seems to be no light at the end of her tunnel.

▼ At eighty-two, Gloria is in good health and should be looking forward to moving into a new, cozy apartment with her husband of sixty years, eighty-three-year-old Paul. Instead she feels empty and numb. The move from the family home has stunned her. At the same time, she's had to cope with her husband's controlling attitude and personality that has become even more severe and unyielding as he's aged. Realizing that it's up to her to organize their lives and make things happen, Gloria feels overwhelmed and defeated.

Four women, all in different stages of life, all from different socioeconomic and psychosocial backgrounds, all with very distinct personalities. Yet they have one thing in common: They suffer from depression, a serious, debilitating medical condition. The illness undermines their health and disrupts their daily lives. If left untreated, depression could lead them to commit suicide: the cause of death of some 3,500 women—most of them depressed—every year.

THE AGE OF MELANCHOLY

Depression is one of the most common health problems in the United States today. According to the National

Institute of Mental Health, more than 1 in 20 Americans—some 17.8 million people—suffer depression every year. Women become depressed about twice as often as men, which makes the disorder one of the most gender-specific of all psychological problems.

Depression is an expensive illness, costing the American economy about $44 million in lost work days, poor performance on the job, psychotherapeutic care, and loss of lifetime earnings due to suicide every year. Its personal cost is incalculable. It is a disease that robs the spirit of life and the body of energy. Measured by days spent in bed and body pain experienced, depression ranks second only to advanced heart disease in exacting a physical toll. Those who have known its relentlessly oppressive nature speak of it as a kind of living death, a deep darkness of the soul. F. Scott Fitzgerald, who suffered depression along with his wife Zelda, described the illness this way: "In a real dark night of the soul it is always three o'clock in the morning, day after day." In this nocturnal void, the self wages an intimate struggle against hopelessness and despair.

Yet as intensely personal and internal as depression may seem, its effects spread beyond the individual into the circle of family, friends, and work relationships. A study published in a 1989 issue of the *Journal of the American Medical Association* reported that depression is more isolating and socially devastating than any other chronic illness. As the joy in living dissipates, a depressed person pushes away the warm blanket of companionship and intimacy, often leaving the people in her life to feel as cold, alone, and helpless as she does. In fact, according to another study, more than 40 percent of people living with a depressed person require some psychological help to cope with their own lives and emotional problems, and about one in five spouses of depressed people become depressed themselves.

Chances are, you've picked up this book because you're

concerned that you or someone close to you may be suffering from depression. By doing so, you've taken the first—and perhaps most difficult—step toward recovery. It is an act of courage not everyone has the strength or foresight to take. According to the National Institute of Mental Health, fewer than one in every three depressed people ever seek treatment. As we'll discuss further in chapter 2, there remains a great deal of shame and guilt associated with mental illness that too often keeps people from seeking the help they need.

The good news—the news you should take to heart—is that more than 80 percent of those people who do seek treatment experience significant improvement in just a few months. In recent years, scientists have learned a great deal about the human brain and its circuitry, and this knowledge has led to the development of more effective treatment options.

We've designed this book to help women with depression understand their illness and find the help they need to get well. Although women appear to be more vulnerable to depression than men, we also seem to be better equipped to handle such an emotional and physical crisis. On average, we tend to live longer than men and are far less likely to succeed in ending our lives by suicide than our male counterparts. We can talk to each other and to our doctors with more ease and openness, and can thus reach out for help before it's too late.

Nevertheless, depression remains a growing health concern for both sexes. As we head into the twenty-first century, depressive illness has become more and more common for both men and women. One study found that people born during the 1950s are a remarkable *twenty times* more likely to suffer a bout of depression than people born during the 1920s. No doubt part of the reason for this increase is that the media has helped spread the word about depression and its symptoms, leading more people to identify depression as the cause of their physical and mental problems.

But that's just a small part of the picture. Many sociologists and psychologists believe that the last several decades of dramatic social change have left modern men and women particularly vulnerable to mood disorders like depression. Family life has disintegrated to the point where we no longer can count on the kind of emotional support that our parents and grandparents received within the family. The influences of religious, moral, and cultural traditions have waned, too, along with our trust in social structures like the government and educational institutions. Cynicism has largely replaced patriotism in the national psyche.

This social disintegration has left us feeling isolated and alone, which is ripe enough ground for feelings of depression to take root. In addition, because we feel too much as if we're struggling only for ourselves and not for the greater good of family or community, our failures seem all the more personal and devastating, even relatively minor ones like losing a job or ending a romantic relationship. Taken together with the fact that most of us were brought up to expect more from life—higher living standards, more material goods, increased professional success, better mental and physical health—than our parents, this emphasis on the self and self-realization may end up overwhelming and defeating us rather than spurring us on to achievement.

THE FEMALE FACTOR

Presumably this burden of isolation, self-involvement, and potential for profound disappointment falls equally upon

men and women. Why, then, do so many more women
than men become depressed? Most researchers now agree
that a woman's physiology, so closely regulated by hormonal fluctuations, is one key to understanding this phe-
nomenon. Indeed, depression in women is often triggered
by biological events, such as the onset of puberty, monthly
menstruation, giving birth, and the onset of menopause.

Far more than is true for men, powerful hormones direct the course of our lives, influencing our behavior as
well as our health in complex ways still not completely understood by medical science. Without a doubt, hormones
and psychosocial factors combine to make women more
vulnerable than men to depression. Yet there remains
some resistance to the idea that biological imperatives
could affect a woman's mental health. One reason for this
is that these same hormonal events are also laden with
sociological and personal considerations: the onset of puberty, for instance, carries with it the awareness of sexuality with all of its confusing signals and social changes.
Often upsetting questions regarding body image—a major
factor in the development of a woman's self-esteem—and
future societal roles come into play at this time as well. As
menopause approaches, hormonal changes coexist with
other signs of aging, with the loss of fertility, and with the
specter of old age and dying. The psychosocial issues that
surround these biological events, some say, may be just as
responsible for triggering depression as any concurrent
surge or depletion of hormones.

Another reason for shying away from a biological explanation for the high rates of depression among women is
a political one. Blaming a serious mental health problem
on unavoidable biological functions, this thinking goes,
harkens back to the antiquated notion of the female as the
weaker and intrinsically more emotional gender. If biology
is destiny, then how can we compete on an equal basis with

men, who apparently have fewer hormonally related health issues to consider? In the past, justified fears of further discrimination against women have prevented some scientists from following avenues of research involving biological influences on depression. Fortunately, more objective and comprehensive studies of women's health in general, and of women and depression in particular, are taking place in laboratories here in the United States and around the world.

Without question, however, several social factors also contribute to our greater risk for developing depression. One theory is that men and women are raised to respond differently to the same stimuli. Generally speaking, men are brought up to be more aggressive and better able to express anger than women. Women tend to react rather than to act, and to focus more on relationships with others as a source of happiness and self-esteem than do men. Women are also more likely to blame and punish themselves, even for events over which they have no control. Men, on the other hand, tend to respond to frustration and disappointment by acting with violence and substance abuse rather than with introspection and depression. In other words, men are more likely to explode rather than implode when faced with stress.

Interestingly, similar patterns of chemical imbalances in the brain often occur with violence, substance abuse, and depression, specifically, a disruption in the level of a neurotransmitter called serotonin. That means that stress causes very similar changes in brain chemistry in both men and women, but we react differently to these changes based on the way we've been brought up in this gender-biased society. This would help to explain why rates for both violence among men and depression among women have steadily climbed, apparently in tandem, during the late twentieth century.

Furthermore, violence in this society too often is perpetrated by men against women, and too often by men presumed to love the women they abuse. According to statistics compiled by the Federal Bureau of Investigation, a woman is battered every 15 seconds by an intimate partner. Sexual abuse is just as common. According to the American Psychological Association Special Task Force on Women and Depression, a shocking 37 percent of women have a significant experience of physical or sexual abuse before the age of twenty-one. As we'll discuss later, each individual woman who suffers this kind of victimization runs a higher risk of developing depression, both while enduring the abuse and later, as a symptom of posttraumatic stress disorder. At the same time, the societal level of violence affects the entire female gender. We feel less secure, less able to trust our own instincts, less in control of our destinies—at least in terms of violence—than our male counterparts, and thus perhaps more susceptible to mood disorders like depression.

Other social factors also influence the high rates of depression in women. Although the status of women in society in general, and in the workplace in particular, has risen during the past few decades, women still earn less than men for the same work, suffer more discrimination and harassment, and the work they do remains, on the whole, less valued than "men's work." Historically, studies have shown that women who stay at home tend to suffer the highest rates of depression, partly because housework and childcare are undervalued and partly because they are apt to be boring and repetitive. The women who are least likely to become depressed are wives and mothers who also hold *part-time,* paid jobs outside the home. Although long-range studies have yet to be done, it is likely that the pressures on those who attempt to "have it all"—to be mothers and wives and full-time employees outside the home—may leave women just as vulnerable to depression as their single-role sisters.

In the end, the sociological reasons why so many Americans, and American women in particular, seem to be depressed these days may be impossible to identify with any degree of certainty. As discussed, scientists have discovered that brain chemistry and other biological factors have far more to do with an individual's risk of developing depression—and her ability to get well—than any combination of social factors. Although the stress of twentieth century living may help to trigger depression in vulnerable people, it is not the only factor.

"It took me a long time to get help because I thought it wasn't anything about *me* but about the world around me that was making me so miserable," remarks Beth. "Who wouldn't be depressed with the amount of violence in our society? Who wouldn't lack energy if no matter how hard you pedaled, you ended up in the same place on the road? What I didn't realize for the longest time was that something inside of my brain, my body, was causing my symptoms, something that medicine and therapy could help. I didn't have to wait around for society to change. I could make myself whole again, and then change my life."

UNDERSTANDING DEPRESSION

Defining depression is not an easy task, since the condition tends to affect everyone in a slightly different way. In fact, it may be easier to describe what depression is *not* rather than what it is: It isn't "the blues" or feeling low for a few hours or even for several days. It isn't the sadness that comes after a relationship breaks up, or the drop in self-esteem that occurs after being fired from a job or failing to meet a goal. Depression is not grief, not even deep grief that envelops and suffocates with its intensity. It isn't a bad mood or feeling consistently grouchy or out-of-sorts.

Instead, depression is a whole body illness, involving changes in body chemistry that cause a variety of symptoms. Depression affects not just your emotions, but also your physical health and the way you think and behave. One of the reasons that depression so often goes undiagnosed is that some people remain unaware that their problems could be related to a mood disorder.

There are three primary categories of depression: major depression, *dysthymia,* and *bipolar disorder.* Major depression is a disorder that significantly alters behavior and health, often interfering with the ability to manage daily life. In its most severe form, it may require psychiatric hospitalization for a period of time. Dysthymia, or chronic mild depression, tends to have milder symptoms than major depression, but also can be longer lasting. Whether or not dysthymia is a separate entity from major depression or simply a less intense version of the same disorder remains a subject of debate. Finally, bipolar disorder involves periods of manic (high strung, high energy) behavior followed by periods of depression. Probably the most serious of depressive disorders, bipolar disorder requires both pharmacologic (drug) treatment and therapeutic intervention. At times, bipolar disorder can cause a psychiatric emergency requiring recurrent psychiatric hospitalization.

In addition, there exist several other subcategories of depression, each with its own set of symptoms and possible triggers.

▼ *Seasonal affective disorder (SAD)* involves periods of depression on an annual basis during the same time each year—beginning most often between the months of October and November as the days grow shorter and ending in

March or April with the coming of spring. The National Institute of Mental Health estimates that about ten million Americans suffer with SAD, most of them in the northern part of the country where it stays darker longest.

▼ *Premenstrual dysphoric disorder (PMDD)* is related to premenstrual syndrome. PMDD occurs in an estimated 1 to 3 percent of all menstruating women, who experience symptoms of depression during the last week of their menstrual cycles and cannot function as usual at work, home, or school.

▼ *Postpartum depression* affects about 1 percent of all new mothers, usually within four weeks after delivering their babies, though it can occur any time within the first year.

We discuss the similarities and differences among the various types of depression further in chapters 2 and 3.

THE SYMPTOMS OF DEPRESSION

"Numb," says Marilyn. "That's the only word I can think of to describe how I feel sometimes." Gail describes her condition as "a kind of viselike bad mood that makes me feel nervous and stuck at the same time." "Like a heavy wet blanket," claims Beth. Gloria talks about depression as feeling "like someone comes in and drains the blood right out of me."

As you can see from just these four women, depression feels different to every person who experiences it. There are, however, a wide variety of common symptoms that together define depression, and they involve our emotions, thought processes, behavior, and physical health.

Somatic Disturbances

Headaches, stomach problems, insomnia, loss of appetite, changes in menstruation . . . the list of physical complaints related to depression is extensive and often overlooked as symptoms of a psychological disorder. In fact, most people with depression first visit a doctor complaining not of emotional problems but of physical ones. As we discuss further in chapter 3, the physician may recognize the underlying depression or may not. Hopefully, the physician will know what questions to ask and will be able to identify the symptoms of depression. Otherwise, women may undergo unnecessary tests and treatments, only to end up feeling just as sick.

The most common—and often the first—symptom of depression tends to involve a change in sleep patterns. Many women with depression suffer from insomnia (the inability to get and stay asleep), hypersomnia (sleeping much more than usual), or early wakening (several hours earlier than normal). Another physical symptom is fatigue, a lack of energy and motivation that can be overwhelming. In other cases, depressed women report feeling more agitated and irritable than usual, pacing and fidgeting rather than feeling lethargic. Another common somatic complaint is gastrointestinal disorder, especially irritable bowel syndrome. Research suggests that up to 40 percent of all cases of irritable bowel syndrome may be caused by depression.

Changes in eating habits also occur in severe depression. In most cases, depressed women lose their appetite and hence begin to lose weight. In a significant minority, however, the opposite is true. Gail, for instance, ends every day sitting on the couch, watching television as the baby sleeps, eating potato chips, one after another in a kind of nervous frenzy, until she's consumed a whole bag. "I feel like such a failure, on top of everything else, for having gained all this weight," Gail complains. "I keep thinking eating will calm me down, make me feel better, but of course it doesn't. I just feel lazy and out of control. I feel terrible because I don't think I attract my husband anymore."

Some symptoms of depression are so far afield that they're often missed. For example, increasing evidence suggests that depression may impede a woman's fertility. That is according to psychologist Alice Domar, director of the Mind/Body Center for Women's Health and the Infertility Program at Beth Israel Deaconess Medical Center in Boston. In 1998, Domar announced that 44 percent of 174 chronically infertile patients who completed her 10-week stress-reduction workshop became pregnant within six months.

Emotional Changes

Perhaps the most obvious impact depression makes is on our feelings and our moods. Sadness is the most common feeling, and tearfulness its frequent expression. "Mornings have always been the most difficult for me," Beth admits, "but the truth is, I find myself crying at the oddest times. All of a sudden, while I'm making my lunch or starting the car or brushing my hair, my eyes just flood with tears and my heart just starts to break. I don't even know what brings it on most of the time."

But sadness is just one aspect of depression's emotional spectrum. The disorder can trigger a host of other feelings, including:

▼ *Emptiness:* A number of people with depression feel not sad nor desperate, but empty and unconnected to the world. Nothing gives them pleasure, not even favorite activities or beloved friends. Gloria used to look forward to shopping with her daughter every Friday. Today, she goes only if her daughter insists. "I just go through the motions," Gloria admits. "I try as hard as I can to smile and laugh, just so my daughter won't worry. Inside, though, I feel nothing. Not happy, not sad. Just there."

▼ *Hopelessness:* One reason so few people suffering from depression reach out for help is that they truly believe that nothing in the world could change their mood or their situation. The present is unbearable and, in their minds, the future can only get worse.

▼ *Remorse:* And if the future looks bleak to someone who is depressed, the past is a place filled with disappointment, darkness, and regret. "I get stuck in the past so much," Beth says, "and all I see is where I went wrong. Leaving my career to care for the kids, wrecking my marriage, it's all my fault when I'm like this. There's a part of me that knows it isn't true, that *I'm* not all bad, but I can't seem to get past this. It's how I feel."

▼ *Guilt:* Sometimes depression brings on a debilitating cycle of diminished activity followed by anxiety and then guilt. Lacking energy and motivation, many depressed people fail to perform regular chores, fall behind at work, or neglect the people closest to them. This creates tension and stress, more reasons to feel like an unworthy failure. "I know I'm not taking care of my baby the way I should," claims Gail, "and that makes me feel even worse. I get all tense and anxious as soon as I wake up, just knowing I'm failing at the one thing I'm supposed to be good at, the one thing I've always wanted to be: a mother."

Cognitive Changes

Quite apart from emotional changes, depression interferes with our ability to think clearly. Because we so rarely equate faulty memory or poor concentration with depression, these cognitive changes can be particularly worrisome. "Although I felt sad because I broke up with my boyfriend, what really made me scared about my health was the way I couldn't study anymore," Marilyn remembers. "I'd sit in front of my books and just stare. When I did read, I couldn't comprehend anything. I'd have to go over every paragraph two or three times before it would make sense. More often than not, I'd just give up and go to bed."

Many women—and men, for that matter—who become depressed also lose their sex drive. "Sex?" asks Gail. "I don't even think about it. I don't even remember what it was like to feel passion. At first I thought it was just having the baby, but now I'm beginning to think something else is wrong. So is my husband." Lack of libido and the inability to respond sexually, which often includes difficulty becoming aroused or achieving orgasm, often accompany a depression.

Behaviorial Changes

Depression often causes us to change the way we act. Most of the time, a depressed person will withdraw from normal social activity and personal interaction. "Just the thought of having to talk to anyone oppressed me," Gloria admits. "I avoided the phone, canceled my bridge games, didn't even go shopping with my daughter. I just wanted to be alone, all alone."

As you'll see in chapter 2, sorting out these symptoms

to attain a diagnosis of depression is not always an easy task—even for doctors trained to do just that. Not only do somatic complaints often mask depression, but many physical illnesses cause symptoms that resemble depression. Doctors must rule out these conditions before treating a patient for a mood disorder. Another complication involves the fact that depression often coexists with other psychological disorders. Gail, for instance, suffers with a concurrent anxiety disorder, while Marilyn struggles with an eating disorder as yet undisclosed even to her new therapist.

Do you recognize yourself in any of these women? Are you plagued by one or more of the symptoms described above? If so, you may be suffering from depression. And you're not alone. As stated at the beginning of the chapter, depression affects nearly eighteen million men, women, and children every year.

THE DEMOGRAPHICS OF DEPRESSION

Depression does not discriminate: The disorder affects people of every age, race, religion, and culture. Although each one of us has a specific set of genetic, social, and personal qualities that puts us at greater or lesser risk of becoming depressed, there are some general categories of people who appear to be at significantly higher risk than the average population. Among the factors that raise the risk are a family history of depression (or other psychological problems), age, and gender.

Heredity

Like many other physical and psychological disorders, depression often runs in families. Although researchers have not yet identified the specific gene involved, studies show that relatives of people who have depression have an overall two to three times higher risk of developing the disease than people without a family history. A child with one depressed parent has a 26 percent higher risk than the rest of the population; with two depressed parents, the risk increases to about 46 percent.

As you might expect, the genetic connection is strongest between identical twins brought up together in the same family. If one identical twin becomes depressed, the other runs about a 76 percent chance of developing the disorder. Even if the twins are raised separately, the concordance rate—the rate of similarity—is about 67 percent. This statistic points to the strong genetic component involved in the development of depression.

Does this mean that if you are or have been depressed that your children are doomed to inherit the disorder from you? Not necessarily. It only means that their *risk* of depression is higher than someone without a family history. Clearly, environmental and psychological factors also come into play when it comes to a complex disorder like depression. But by understanding your family's genetic vulnerability, and by watching carefully for early signs of depression in you and your children, you may be able to get help before a depressive disorder has a chance to take hold.

Age

Depression recognizes no age barrier. Young children, teenagers, and men and women of all ages develop depression. Although depression among children appears to be on the increase, it is still relatively rare. Only about 1 percent of young children develop the disorder, and that percentage is equally divided between boys and girls.

As children enter puberty, however, more and more of them become depressed. About 5 percent of adolescents develop major depression and an additional 3.5 percent suffer from chronic mild depression (dysthymia). It is at this point that the differences in rates between men and women start to diverge, with more adolescent girls than boys becoming depressed. By the time girls hit their late teens, they're at particularly high risk, according to a 1999 UCLA study that found that fully 47 percent of a group of girls experienced one or more episodes of major clinical depression within five years after graduating from high school and moving onto college. Unfortunately, depression in adolescents is often masked by other problems, ranging from learning disabilities to eating disorders to substance abuse. And depression in this age group can be highly lethal if left untreated: An estimated 5,000 adolescents kill themselves in the United States each year, and another 400,000 make unsuccessful attempts annually. In fact, suicide is the third leading cause of death in adolescents.

The most vulnerable age group for depression in both men and women is between the ages of twenty-five and forty-four. About one in four women and one in ten men in this age group will develop depression. The average age when a person first becomes depressed is between twenty to twenty-two years old. During the last few decades, the average age for experiencing a first episode of depression has decreased from about age thirty to about age twenty. By age twenty-five, about 10 percent of this age group may have already experienced at least one bout of depression. After age forty-four or so, depression rates tend to level off.

Contrary to popular belief, old age does not mean automatic melancholy. Just the opposite is true: Healthy, independent men and women over the age of sixty-five experience less depression, on average, than younger adults. However, one sector of this population runs a greater risk than others: Perhaps as many as 28 percent of nursing home residents have symptoms of major depression due to the combination of increased isolation and severe illness.

Diagnosing and treating depression in the elderly can be complicated by many factors. Some illnesses common among the elderly, such as heart disease and chronic conditions like arthritis and Alzheimer's disease, can trigger depression while at the same time masking its symptoms. Both physicians and family members tend to be too quick to attribute depressive symptoms to medical problems or as a simple fact of aging. In fact, a National Institutes of Health panel warned that more than 60 percent of older Americans suffering from depression are not receiving appropriate therapy.

"Even my daughter was quick to say that maybe my 'bad mood' was an appropriate response to the fact that I'm getting older, that my life is almost finished," Gloria remarks. "I guess we all kind of expect old people to be sad and depressed. I'm finding out, though, that there's no need for me to feel this way."

Gender

As discussed, women are two to three times more likely than men to develop major depression, dysthymia, and seasonal affective disorder. According to the *Diagnostic and Statistical Manual of Mental Disorders (DSM-IV)*, the manual of the American Psychiatric Association, a woman's lifetime risk for major depression ranges from 10 to 25 percent, compared with 5 to 12 percent for men. We've already talked about some of the biological and psychosocial reasons for this gender difference in depression rates, and we'll continue this discussion in the chapters that follow.

HERE COMES THE SUN

Studying the epidemiological aspects of a disease—identifying who in the population it most affects and why—can help scientists narrow down its cause. We know a lot about the "who" of depression. Women get depressed more often than men, the disease tends to first strike young adults between the ages of twenty and forty-four, and relatives of people with depression are more likely to become depressed than those without a family history.

The "why" of depression, however, is more elusive. Why is Gail depressed when her sister, brought up in the same household and subject to the same pressures as the mother of a five-year-old daughter, is not? Why do some women suffer postpartum depression or depression related to premenstrual syndrome while other women seem to sail through these biological events? Why is one family plagued with bipolar disorder or major depression while a family living right next door and dealing with the same psychosocial stresses escapes mental illness altogether?

Despite the fact that depression and other types of mental illness have been part of the human experience since the dawn of time, we still don't know the answers to these questions. One reason is that Western medical science has tried to keep separate the body and the mind, resisting the idea that biology could affect emotions and vice versa. Well into the twentieth century, the general public and medical professionals alike considered mental illnesses to be due to problems of character and upbringing rather than to body chemistry or other organic influences.

The good news is that that approach led to the development of different types of psychotherapy, which have helped people come to terms and work through many emotional problems. However, it eventually became clear that there was more to the story of the brain than met the eye—even the trained professional eye—and that psychotherapy might not be the only or total solution for many people suffering from mental illness.

During the 1950s, scientists discovered what many had suspected for some time: mental disorders could be treated with medication. The first breakthrough involved the drug chlorpromazine (Thorazine), which doctors developed to treat schizophrenia. The fact that chemicals could help to restore mental functioning in people once racked with delusions and hallucinations meant that more than personal weakness or emotional trauma lay at the heart of this serious mental disorder—and perhaps many other disorders as well. Soon after, scientists synthesized tranquilizers to help treat psychosis and paranoia, and antidepressants to lift the moods of those depressed. In 1970, the drug known as lithium helped bring balance to those who suffered the wild mood swings of bipolar disorder.

Our understanding of the interconnections among body, mind, and spirit deepened with the development of sophisticated scanning instruments during the 1970s and

1980s. Today, the CT and the MRI scans allow us to map the brain's chemical and electrical activity so that we can actually witness manifestations of thought processes and emotional reactions as they take place. In this way, we can begin to trace both healthy and unhealthy patterns and thus understand even more about the causes and course of depression and other mental problems.

As we head toward the twenty-first century, then, there is much good news for people with, or at risk for, depression. Scientists continue to develop new medications that address depression more effectively and with fewer side effects. We're learning more about how hormonal changes and other natural cycles—including how much we sleep and how much light we are exposed to—affect our moods on a daily, seasonal, and annual basis. Psychotherapy is becoming ever more tailored to address the specific needs of individuals, couples, families, and even groups of colleagues.

In the next chapter, you'll find out how depression is diagnosed today, as well as discover how many different physical and psychological aspects there are to this complicated mood disorder.

IMPORTANT QUESTIONS AND ANSWERS ABOUT CHAPTER 1

Q. I've heard that girls start suffering from low self-esteem at about age ten and that sociologists think maybe it has something to do with the way teachers treat girls versus boys in the classroom. If that's true, could that attitude affect the high rates of depression seen in adolescent girls?

A. Although we as a society have certainly opened up many social, economic, and educational doors to our daughters, there remains an underlying—sometimes subtle, sometimes overt—gender bias in America today. For instance, studies show that teachers tend to give more weight to the answers boys give in class than those that girls give, especially in subjects like math and science. This bias (which is often expressed very subtly) leads boys and girls to form different self-concepts and hold different expectations for themselves and from the world that they will enter as adults.

There is no question that low self-esteem is a symptom of depression, and often a trigger of the disorder as well. Whether or not fewer girls and women develop depression as the barriers to our success and self-fulfillment come down remains to be seen.

Q. Both depression and eating disorders are seen much more in women than in men. Are they related?

A. As you'll see in chapter 2, eating disorders and depression are common comorbid conditions, which means that they often occur together in the same individual, and often at the same time. Scientists have found that a lack of a neurochemical transmitter called serotonin may be involved in both depression and eating disorders. Furthermore, both eating disorders and depression may be triggered by a combination of poor self-esteem, a tendency toward perfectionism, and distorted images of one's body. In any case, both conditions must be treated or a relapse of one or the other (or both) is bound to occur.

Q. I know this book is about women and depression, but after reading about the symptoms, I'm wondering if my husband might be depressed. Are symptoms different for men?

A. Generally speaking, no. Symptoms of disturbed sleep, feelings of hopelessness and sadness, and changes in appetite are common in both men and women who are depressed. Women, however, are more likely to suffer somatic symptoms (aches and pains, gastrointestinal distress, headaches, etc.) while men tend to act out with aggression or substance abuse. Men may also withdraw from personal contact and retreat into work or athletics rather than express their feelings to the people in their lives.

2

▼

SORTING OUT THE BLUES

Symptoms and Risk Factors

Do you feel sad, hopeless, or empty every day?
Do activities that once gave you pleasure no longer interest you?

Have you lost or gained weight without consciously changing your eating habits?

Are you sleeping much less or more than usual?

Do you seem to act and think more slowly or quickly than you have in the past?

Are you tired or lacking energy?

Do you feel ill, as if there's something wrong with your body?

Would you describe yourself as being worthless and do you feel excessive guilt about past or present behavior?

Is it especially difficult for you to concentrate or make decisions?

Do you have recurrent thoughts about death and/or suicide?

Are you unable to function as you once did, socially, at work, or within the family?

Think about how you've answered these questions. How many symptoms are you experiencing now? Have many of them affected you daily, or almost daily, for two weeks or more? If so, you may not be just ill with "a touch of the flu," or simply under a lot of stress, or exhausted from too much stimulation, or bored by not enough. All of these things could also be true, but the fact is that if you answered yes to many of the preceding questions, you're probably suffering with major depression or dysthymia as well.

At the same time, you shouldn't be too quick to presume that a lingering bad mood or a longer-than-usual recovery time after an illness, loss, or trauma means that you have a psychiatric disorder. Feeling discouraged, lonely, unmotivated, sad, or completely empty is a perfectly normal part of the human experience. Even persistent pessimism—defined by *Webster's New World Dictionary* as "the belief that the existing world is the worst possible . . . that the evil in life outweighs the good"—does not constitute a medical illness, but rather a personal outlook on life, however negative and discouraged. In fact, some people feel that "expecting the worst" is the most appropriate response to an often unfair and difficult life. Writer and humorist Ambrose Bierce once defined a pessimist as "someone who sees the world as it is."

A depressive disorder, on the other hand, is a medical illness that requires treatment. Over a period of time, these feelings can take on a life of their own, causing physical and emotional symptoms that constitute an illness. In this chapter, we outline the criteria by which we define depression in its various forms. As discussed in chapter 1, depression is a physical as well as emotional condition, involving one's whole body, mind, and soul. The questions listed above should help to clarify this issue for you. If you've answered more than three or four of them with a "yes," something is clearly compromising your daily life and general health.

Here's one more question to consider: Have you seen a doctor about your symptoms or mentioned to your physician that you might be depressed? If you haven't, you're not alone. The vast majority of depressed people never seek the help they need to get well. Of those who visit a doctor about their symptoms, most never mention the possibility that their problems could be psychological in origin even if, deep down, they suspect it themselves.

Peri, a forty-three-year-old legal secretary, resisted getting help for several months, despite the fact that she could barely function in her daily life. "I was just starting a new relationship. I thought my periods of panic and sadness were about my fears of commitment, or maybe something about my boyfriend, Jeff. It wasn't until I started remembering things from my past—disturbing things about my childhood that I couldn't deal with—that I talked to my doctor about it."

THE ROOTS OF DENIAL

Why do so many people resist the idea that a mental illness could be at the root of their problems? There are several common reasons, both cultural and personal. See if you might be holding back for any of the following attitudes:

Disbelief

Like Peri, many women simply assume that their problems are circumstantial in origin (a bad marriage, a stressful

job, a tenuous new relationship). Others, like Marilyn, the
college student you met in the first chapter, believe that
their lethargy, difficulty with concentration, and other
symptoms are due to a physical illness. Are you waiting for
your life to change, or for aspirin or rest to alleviate your
symptoms, instead of seeking the help you need?

Shame

Despite the fact that Prozac and other antidepressants are
among the most prescribed drugs in the United States—
which means that millions of men and women take them
because they are depressed—depression and other mental
illnesses still exist behind a shroud of fear and shame.
Perhaps it goes back to the days when the mentally ill were
thought to be possessed by the devil or were shut away in
unpleasant and poorly run institutions without possibility
of cure. Or the blame might be better placed on the continuing false impression that a weakness of character
rather than a medical illness causes mental and emotional
disturbances. Whatever the reasons, many people still feel
too ashamed of themselves, their symptoms, and their behavior to seek treatment for depression. Are you one of
them?

Guilt

Guilt is one of the most isolating and paralyzing of all
emotions, and depression and guilt often travel hand in
hand. One reason for this unfortunate pairing is that people who become depressed shut down both emotionally
and physically. Eventually, the inability to function undermines work, family, and social relationships and responsi-

bilities. This results in a vicious cycle of depression, guilt over failing to meet expectations, followed by more depression. Guilt comes, too, from feeling that somehow you should be able to lift yourself out of depression by simply "pulling yourself up by the bootstraps." When you can't, you blame yourself, adding to the tension, guilt, and disappointment—and further paralyzing you from taking action.

Fear of Rejection

Are you afraid that your friends or colleagues will shun you if you admit you're having trouble? "I wasn't only ashamed, I was also *afraid* to let anyone know how I was feeling," admits Gail, a thirty-two-year-old mother of a young son. "I thought my husband and friends would leave me if they knew the darkness and panic that flooded my brain, or think I was just plain crazy and put me away. It wasn't until I started talking about it that I realized I wasn't alone. So many of my friends had experienced these same feelings, and my husband's brother had required hospitalization for depression once." Because she had been so afraid of being rejected, Gail needlessly put off seeking treatment—and receiving comfort—for several painful and isolating months.

Another fear—fear of being fired or passed over for promotion at work—keeps many people from admitting they have an emotional or mental problem. If worry about your job is holding you back, you should be aware that the 1990 Americans with Disabilities Act offers legal protection to those suffering with major depression, bipolar disorder, and other mental illnesses. The law states that you are under no obligation to tell your employer that you are depressed or receiving treatment for it. Furthermore, at least technically, simply having a mental illness like depression and receiving psychiatric treatment for it is not grounds for dismissal—as long as you're performing the duties of your job.

Unfortunately, in the real world your fears of rejection and discrimination may not be completely unwarranted. There remains a great deal of misinformation about mental illnesses like depression and you may very well face some skepticism at work or in your personal life. Only you—with help from your doctor or therapist—can decide how and when to let people know (a subject we'll discuss at more length in chapter 7).

Helplessness

The very nature of depression is responsible for the number one reason people fail to seek treatment: You may feel so hopeless and helpless that you simply don't have the energy or the will to pick up the phone and make an appointment. "At my worst," Peri admits, "I figured, what's the use? Nothing will get better; there's nothing anyone can do. My sister was the one who finally got me to call a doctor—and she had to stand there while I dialed. But just the act of making an appointment made me feel better. I'm just sorry I waited so long."

Fortunately, there's lots of help out there, in the form of therapists, medical professionals, and support groups. In the next section, we outline the various roles of those professionals to help you choose whom to see first about your problem.

GETTING HELP

Today, you have more choices than ever when it comes to getting help for depression. Well-trained general practitioners, psychiatrists, psychologists, social workers, and therapists are all qualified to diagnose and treat depression. However, each category of professionals has its own distinct advantages and disadvantages. Let's look at them one by one.

Primary Care Physicians

Your primary care physician, otherwise known as your "regular doctor," is probably a specialist in either family practice or internal medicine. Both types of doctors are thoroughly trained in all aspects of medicine, including psychiatric disorders. They can prescribe antidepressants and other drugs, and may also be able to offer you some counseling. If you've been seeing your personal physician for some time, you may feel more comfortable talking about your problems to him or her, at least at first.

You should be aware, though, that not all primary care physicians are on the lookout for psychological explanations for their patients' symptoms. In one study, 51 percent of physicians failed to diagnose depression in their depressed patients. If the patients came in to the office complaining of somatic symptoms, such as headaches or stomachaches, and denied any emotional problem, doctors recognized depression in only 20 percent of the depressed patients. Primary care physicians were more likely to accurately diagnosis depression when patients were willing to accept the idea that their symptoms might be psychological in origin when asked. If you're visiting your doctor with the idea you might be depressed, you may fare better by being upfront about it.

Nevertheless, no matter how comfortable you are with your primary physician, you may decide to seek help from a professional specially trained in mental and emotional problems. If your depression is complicated by another mental disorder such as anxiety, or if you have underlying and recurrent psychosocial issues, you may require more intensive interpersonal counseling than your physician is able to provide. In that case, a psychiatrist, psychologist, or other mental health professional may be your best bet. More than likely your doctor will be glad to recommend further treatment he or she feels is right for you.

Psychiatrists

Psychiatrists are medical doctors who specialize in the diagnosis and treatment of mental or psychiatric disorders. They have completed medical school, a year-long internship, and a three-year residency program that provides training in diagnosis and treatment of psychiatric disorders. They can prescribe medications and make medical decisions.

Psychologists

Psychologists have completed a graduate program in human psychology that includes clinical training and internships in counseling, psychotherapy, and psychological testing. Although most have a doctorate degree (either a Ph.D. or Psy.D.), psychologists have not studied medicine nor can they prescribe medication. Most states require that psychologists be licensed in order to practice independently.

Social Workers

Certified social workers (C.S.W.s) or licensed clinical social workers (L.C.S.W.s) have completed a two-year graduate program with specialized training in helping people with mental problems, in addition to conventional social work. Most states certify or license social workers and require the passage of a qualifying exam.

Psychiatric Nurses

These health care professionals have earned nursing degrees, and have special training and experience in mental health care. No special licensing or certification requirements currently exists for this category of therapists.

The term "therapist" is used to describe almost anyone who helps people cope with mental and emotional problems, from board-certified psychiatrists to licensed psychologists to unlicensed (and largely unregulated) marriage counselors, hypnotherapists, and stress management specialists. Many of these people are highly trained professionals, but others are not. That's why it's important to check references carefully before undergoing treatment with any health care provider. (For the purposes of this book, we'll use the words "doctor," "therapist," and "counselor" interchangeably to refer to the person who treats your depression.)

In chapter 6, we'll discuss finding a good therapist, and how to establish and maintain a good working relationship with him or her. We'll provide some tips and guidelines to help you through the process. In the meantime, you need to take the first important step toward recovery: attaining an accurate assessment of your problem.

DIAGNOSING DEPRESSION

Unlike the process involved in diagnosing most physical illnesses, there exist no blood, urine, or X-ray tests that will confirm or rule out depression. Instead your doctor or therapist makes a diagnosis by interpreting your symptoms and comparing them to a standard set of criteria. Most clinicians use the criteria outlined in a text called *The Diagnostic and Statistical Manual of Mental Disorders,* as well as supplement the process with other tests. Now in its fourth revision, the *DSM-IV,* as it's commonly known, has been the bible of psychiatric diagnosis since it was first published in 1952. The *DSM-IV* organizes symptoms according to disorder, taking away some—but far from all—of the once arbitrary process of psychiatric diagnosis.

As helpful as the *DSM-IV* is to therapists in making a diagnosis, it continues to have some drawbacks. One of its main disadvantages involves a relative exclusion of possible physical causes of symptoms. As we mentioned in chapter 1, modern medicine continues to divide the body from the mind, the physical from the mental and emotional. If you go to your primary physician complaining of sleeplessness, lack of appetite, and lethargy, he or she is more likely to relate those symptoms to a physical illness. If, on the other hand, the first medical stop you make is to a psychiatrist, he or she is more likely to use the *DSM-IV* to relate those symptoms to a mental illness like depression.

The problem is that there really isn't a clear division between mind and body. Several physical illnesses either may cause, exacerbate, or, conversely, mask your emotional and mental problems. Indeed, studies show that mental symptoms may precede the physical signs of some diseases by weeks, months, or even years. At the same time, the pain, isolation, and inactivity associated with being ill can become a trigger for depression, a depression that's often overlooked as you and your doctor work on solving the physical problems. Fortunately, more and more primary physicians and psychiatrists are becoming aware of this complexity, and thus make sure to take both psychiatric and physical problems under consideration with their patients' conditions.

The first thing your doctor will do is take an inventory of your symptoms, both physical and psychological. If you're a new patient, he or she will also take your medical and psychological history, and that of your family. This will help identify any patterns of illnesses in your own life or in your genetic makeup. Clearly, it is extremely important for you to be as open and honest with your doctor as possible. The more information you provide, the more accurate the diagnosis is likely to be.

It is extremely important for you to have a complete physical examination—with laboratory blood and urine tests—if you have not had one in recent months. Your therapist will either recommend that you see a primary physician or conduct the physical exam himself or herself if qualified and equipped to do so. This examination will help to rule out any possible underlying physical problems you might have that could cause or exacerbate your depressive symptoms.

What to Rule Out First

A heart attack, a chronic and debilitating illness like arthritis that slowly but surely saps energy and mobility, an addiction to alcohol or cocaine that takes control over one's life.... Doctors know that these conditions, and many others, can trigger a depression in susceptible individuals. At the same time, these very same conditions may themselves cause symptoms that resemble depression, and once the underlying problem is addressed, the depressive symptoms usually disappear. In fact, severe and chronic medical illness is one of the main underlying triggers for depression.

In addition, there is some as yet largely anecdotal evidence that severe or long-term depression could create a biochemical atmosphere in the body that might make us more vulnerable to heart disease, cancer, or a host of other conditions. A report published in the *Journal of the American Medical Association* in 1991 found that patients with major depressive disorders who were admitted to nursing homes had a startling 59 percent greater likelihood of dying in the first year than those who weren't depressed. And how many times have you heard about a widow who falls ill and dies within months after her husband's death, despite having been in perfect health beforehand? Could it be that grief, which may develop into depression in some cases, causes changes in the immune system or another aspect of normal physiology? Or could it be that depression itself leads to unhealthy behavior, such as heavy drinking or failing to take medication, that exacerbates or promotes physical problems? These are questions that scientists are trying hard to answer, as we'll explore in chapter 3.

For now, let's go back to the subject at hand. What kind

of physical complications should you and your physician consider first when evaluating your symptoms of depression? Here are the most common categories.

Prescription Drugs

A number of widely used medications, a list of which follows, have been implicated in episodes of depression. (We discuss alcohol and illicit drug use later in the chapter.) Virtually any medication that slows down body systems or significantly changes body chemistry can cause depressive symptoms. These include drugs used to treat hypertension and heart disease, psychiatric drugs, over-the-counter antihistamines, estrogen, steroids, and many more.

Generally speaking, more women than men develop depressive side effects to medication. Women tend to become more tearful and sad while men more often react with irritation and crankiness. Furthermore, birth control pills, which contain estrogen and progesterone, often produce depressive side effects: As many as 15 percent of women using oral contraceptives have reported mood changes. Estrogen replacement therapy (ERT) during menopause seems to alleviate depression for many women, while causing it in others. Paradoxically, going off ERT may also trigger mood changes.

Medications Associated with Depression
(Talk to your doctor about *whatever* medications you take.)

Anticonvulsants: used to treat seizure disorders like epilepsy
    carbamazepine (Tegretol, Epitol, Atretol)
    phenytoin sodium (Dilantin)

Antihistamines: used to treat colds and allergies
diphenhydramine hydrochloride (Benadryl)
any of a number of over-the-counter drugs

Antihypertensives/Cardiac drugs: used to treat high
blood pressure, angina, and heart attack
clonindine (Catapres)
diltiazem hydrochloride (Cardizem)
guanethidine (Ismelin)
hydralazine (Aspresoline Hydrocloride)
proprandol hydrochloride (Inderal)
resperine (Serpasil, Ser-Ap-Es)

Antiparkinsonism agents
levodopa (Doper, larodopa)
levodopa and carbidopa (Sinemet)
bromocriptine mesylate (Parlodel)

Benzodiazepines: used to treat anxiety disorders
alprazolam (Xanax)
diazepam (Valium)

Corticosteroids: used to treat arthritis and other autoim-
mune diseases, asthma, and cancer, among other conditions
prednisone (Pred Forte, Deltasone, Orasone)
cortisone

Hormones
estrogen
progesterone
discontinuation of estrogen replacement therapy

If your depression is medication-related, it's very likely
that your doctor can help by simply switching you to another drug, one that does not disrupt your body chemistry
in the same way. Usually there are several different options
available, even with birth control pills. If there are no effective alternatives—if you're taking corticosteroids for a
severe and chronic disease like arthritis or multiple sclero-

sis, for instance—then your doctor may decide to pre-scribe an antidepressant for you that will counteract the medication's depressive side effects.

In any case, you can see why it is extremely important to let your doctor or therapist know about all the medication you take. First, many drugs cause depressive symptoms that can usually be alleviated quite simply by changing the drug or lowering its dose. Second, antidepressants may in-teract adversely with other medications, leading to poten-tially dangerous, even fatal, complications.

Endocrine Disorders

The endocrine system—the body system that produces the powerful chemicals called hormones—works in close co-operation with the nervous system. The intimate interac-tion between the two systems means that any disturbance in normal hormone levels can lead to a wide range of neurological and mood changes, including symptoms of depression. In fact, two of the brain's most important neuro-transmitters, norepinephrine and epinephrine, are also hormones produced by the adrenal glands.

Any one of a number of endocrine disorders can pro-duce depressive symptoms, including hypothyroidism, hyper-thyroidism, Cushing's disease, Addison's disease, Wilson's disease, diabetes, hyperparathyroidism, and hypoglycemia. Diabetes mellitus is a good example. This disease involves the failure of the pancreas to produce enough insulin—the hormone that helps the body break down food and convert it into energy—or the failure of body cells to use insulin properly. If left untreated or poorly managed, dia-betes can cause low energy, weakness, irritability, and diffi-culty with concentration—all signs of major depression as well. We've already mentioned the suspected relationship

between the female sex hormones, estrogen and progesterone, and depression.

When it comes to depressive symptoms, perhaps the
most common culprit in the endocrine system is the thyroid gland. Located in the neck below the Adam's apple,
the thyroid gland secretes hormones instrumental in almost all metabolic processes, controlling the rate of metabolism and also the body's consumption of calories. The
hormones stimulate growth, are essential for the normal
development of the central nervous system, and also enhance the action of the adrenal gland's stress hormones
(epinephrine and norepinephrine).

There are two major types of thyroid disease, both more
common in women than men. Sometimes called myx-
edema, hypothyroidism is the clinical term for an underactive thyroid gland. If your thyroid is underactive, your
body processes are slower than usual, leading to feelings of
fatigue or sluggishness, weight gain, slowed thinking, and
dark moods—again, all common symptoms of major depression.

Hyperthyroidism, on the other hand, is an overactive
thyroid, which means that the gland secretes excess hormone and thus speeds up the body's metabolic rate.
Although a far less common mimicker of depression, hyperthyroidism may also have symptoms of irritability,
weight loss, and fatigue.

Central Nervous System Diseases

The brain is the most complex organ in the body, and scientists continue to explore its structure and physiology. By
doing so, they hope to unravel the still fascinating and un-
solved mysteries of memory, thought, personality, behavior, and mood.

In the meantime, we already know a great deal about disorders of the brain that may also cause depressive symptoms. These disorders include Alzheimer's disease, Parkinson's disease, epilepsy, multiple sclerosis, Huntington's chorea, and stroke. Research indicates that depression affects more than 80 percent of people with Alzheimer's disease, a type of dementia that affects about two million Americans, most of them over the age of sixty-five. Often the first and most persistent symptoms of multiple sclerosis (MS), a chronic degenerative disease of the central nervous system, include mood changes such as dips of sadness and/or periods of euphoria that could be mistaken for depression or bipolar disorder. In Parkinson's disease, the neurotransmitter dopamine becomes depleted. Dopamine is one of the brain's most important chemicals because it helps different parts of the brain and body—including those involving mood and emotion—communicate with one another.

Cancer

Cancer is a term used to describe any number of diseases involving abnormal and uncontrolled growth of cells—and almost all of them may trigger depressive symptoms. Depression is often the very first symptom of the fast-growing and nearly always fatal pancreatic cancer. Central nervous system tumors, such as those of the left temporal and frontal lobes of the brain and of the limbic system (deep inside the brain) are also very likely to produce early symptoms of depression and irritability. It should be noted, though, that less than 2 percent of all depressions that are later diagnosed as physical diseases turn out to be cancer.

Heart Disease

It appears that depression is a common side effect of heart attacks, coronary artery disease, and angina (chest pains). A 1994 study published in the British medical journal *Lancet* found that depressed heart attack patients were twice as likely to suffer chest pains than nondepressed patients with the same degree of heart disease. Exactly how and why heart disease itself might cause depression is still unknown, but we do know that medications to treat its symptoms very often have depressive side effects.

Infectious Disease

Many infectious diseases, such as viral pneumonia, hepatitis, tuberculosis, and mononucleosis, can cause a variety of mood disturbances, including symptoms of depression. Chronic fatigue syndrome, an apparently new disease that emerged in the late 1980s, has symptoms that closely resemble depression, including low energy, somatic complaints like headaches and stomachaches, and mood disturbances. Acquired Immune Deficiency Syndrome (AIDS) also may have symptoms related to depression, especially should the disease allow opportunistic infections of the central nervous system to take hold.

As you can see, there is a chance that your symptoms of low self-esteem, lethargy, hopelessness, appetite and sleep changes, and somatic complaints could be signs of a physical illness requiring a very different kind of treatment approach than a classic depression. That's why it's important that you receive a complete physical examination before you and your doctor assume that you are depressed. Once that's been accomplished, and you've ruled out other possible causes, you and your therapist can start to look at your mental and emotional problems with more clarity and direction.

THE TYPES OF DEPRESSION

Depression is a very personal disease. Each woman with depression experiences it just a little differently from everyone else. One person might feel tense and edgy, while another is deadened, numb. Gail sits in her living room, night after night, eating junk food and watching television, while Gloria closes herself off completely, unable to concentrate even on a TV show or to look at food with any appetite. Both Peri and Gail suffer with accompanying anxiety, while Marilyn struggles with an intermittent eating disorder.

Despite the individual nature of depression, however, clinicians have created some general categories of the disease based on when symptoms occur, how long they last, and of what they consist. We mentioned these categories briefly in chapter 1. Now let's look at them in a little more depth.

Major Depression

"There's no point in treating a depressed person as though she were just feeling sad, saying 'There now, hang on, you'll get over it,'" wrote author Barbara Kingsolver in her novel *The Bean Trees*. "Sadness is more or less like a head cold—with patience it passes. Depression is like a cancer."

According to the National Institute of Mental Health, major depression is the single most widespread mental disorder, affecting 10.3 percent of Americans in any given year. It consists of a depressed mood or loss of interest or pleasure in usual activities for a period of two weeks or longer. Its symptoms, which we've already discussed at length in chapter 1, can be mild, moderate, or severe. If you answered yes to just a few of the questions listed at the beginning of this chapter, and are still able to perform most of your activities as usual, you probably have a mild depression. The more symptoms you experience, and the more they interfere with your daily life, the more severe your depression.

Currently, therapists identify three different forms of major depression: melancholic, atypical, and psychotic. Melancholic depression involves symptoms of deep sadness and feelings of slowness and lethargy. The depression with which Beth suffers is a classic case of melancholic depression. Beth wakes before dawn, her symptoms are most severe in the morning then lessen as the day wears on. She has no appetite—for food or for life—and withdraws from social contact as much as possible.

Gail's depression might be classified as atypical. She is more nervous and fraught with anxiety than sad, she's gaining instead of losing weight, and sleeps more rather than less. She's highly conscious of people's opinions of her—especially her husband's—and fears being rejected by her family and friends because of her self-perceived shortcomings. Gail is also troubled by panic disorder, a frequent fellow traveler of depression, as we'll discuss later in the chapter.

The third, and rarest, form of major depression is psychotic depression. In addition to typical depressive symptoms, psychotic depression causes individuals to lose touch with reality and often to experience delusions and hallucinations. Psychotic depression usually requires immediate drug therapy and perhaps hospitalization because its sufferers are unable to function and are at highest risk for suicide. We'll meet a woman with psychotic depression in chapter 4.

Dysthymia

Also known as chronic depression or neurotic depression, dysthymia is defined as a depression in which a person is bothered by depressive symptoms most or all of the time during a period of at least a year. People with dysthymia describe feeling "under a cloud even on a sunny day," "seeing the world as gray and foggy," or "always feeling one stroke below par." The National Comorbidity Survey estimates that about 6.4 percent of Americans develop this disorder at some point in life. Although dysthymia usually develops before the age of twenty-five, most people are not diagnosed until they reach their mid-thirties to early forties or even fifties.

Although the symptoms of dysthymia are similar to depression, they tend to be milder, but longer lasting. Many people with dysthymia claim that they've felt low and depressed for so long they don't remember feeling any other way. Even after treatment, about 5 percent of those with dysthymia never fully recover and remain sad for two years or more after their initial diagnosis. Most, however, can find relief with psychotherapy, medication, or a combination of both.

Dysthymia often coexists with other mental disorders. In fact, the National Institute of Mental Health estimates that about 75 percent of individuals with dysthymia also have periods of major depression (a syndrome called *double depression*), panic disorder, anxiety disorders, or substance abuse. Other studies have linked dysthymia with attention deficit disorder, conduct disorder, and personality disorders.

Seasonal Affective Disorder (SAD)

For millions of people, the arrival of autumn signals not the pleasure associated with the scent of burning leaves or the refreshing crispness of the air, but instead a darkening of spirit, a closing down of the soul. An estimated ten million Americans suffer from seasonal affective disorder, or SAD, and for them, the fall (and less often the spring or summer) is a harbinger of depression.

Emily Dickinson, a poet who lived in Massachusetts—a state known for its spectacular fall foliage and its harsh winters—during the nineteenth century, wrote this poem that cogently sums up SAD's distinctive symptoms:

> *There is a certain slant of light,*
> *Winter afternoons,*
> *That oppresses like the heft*
> *Of cathedral tunes.*
>
> *Heavenly hurt, it gives us.*
> *We can find no scar*
> *But internal difference*
> *Where the meanings are.*

People with SAD usually suffer from the same depressive symptoms as others—feelings of sadness, helplessness, hopelessness, guilt, and mild illness. They tend to eat more than usual during this time, gain weight, and crave rich carbohydrates. They spend many more hours than usual asleep, yet feel chronically exhausted and lethargic. Researchers believe that the amount of sunlight to which we are exposed affects the production and use of body chemicals, including serotonin and norepinephrine, the two neurotransmitters most associated with depression. In addition to benefiting from antidepressant medication and therapy, many people with SAD find treatment with phototherapy (exposure to bright light) extremely helpful in alleviating symptoms.

Premenstrual Dysphoria

Premenstrual syndrome (PMS) is the term given to the group of physical and behavioral changes that affect some women—up to about 70 percent of all those who menstruate—in the week or so before the start of a menstrual period. These symptoms include bloating, fluid retention, weight gain, breast soreness, aching, fatigue, nausea, and headaches, among others. In addition, some women experience emotional changes such as irritability, anxiety, difficulty with concentration, and—for some—depression.

The current version of the *Diagnostic and Statistical Manual of Mental Disorders* identifies a distinct subset of PMS in its section on depression. Called "premenstrual dysphoric disorder" or PMDD, this condition causes about 1 to 3 percent of all menstruating women to experience symptoms of depression during the last week of their menstrual cycles. In most cases, these symptoms resemble those of atypical depression: women with PMDD tend to eat and sleep more than usual and to experience periods of anxiety and mood swings along with feeling sad, discouraged, and hopeless. At times, they may feel paranoid or aggressive, even violent.

Postpartum Depression

"I'm supposed to be happy, but all I feel is sad and anxious," Gail admits. "Just a few weeks after Jeff was born, I started having these feelings that I was unworthy of being a mother, and unable to do anything right. Then came the panic attacks. I know now that I should have gotten help right away, but I was paralyzed when it came to taking care of myself, too."

Like other forms of depression, the kind that grips some women shortly after they give birth feels different to every woman who experiences it. The National Institute of Mental Health estimates that postpartum depression occurs in less than 1 percent of all births, causing sadness, decreased concentration, physical complaints, and feelings of guilt, agitation, and anxiety. Postpartum depression also may trigger obsessive behaviors such as constantly checking on the baby.

For Gail, postpartum depression developed into an almost full-blown panic disorder. "There are days when I simply can't leave the house," Gail admits. "I'm afraid something will happen to the baby, a car will hit the carriage or someone will grab him from me. It's horrible. In my head, I know it isn't true, but I can't seem to open the door and walk out into the sunlight."

Postpartum depression can affect any woman—seemingly out of the blue—but women who have had previous depressive episodes appear more likely to suffer the disorder than those without such a history. Another risk factor is the amount of social and financial support available to the woman after the birth: The more isolated and poor a woman is, the more likely she is to suffer postpartum depression.

Bipolar Disorder

Nearly two million American adults—about one in one hundred—suffer from a bipolar disorder, which is characterized by periods of depression followed by extreme highs, or mania. The various types of bipolar illness account for about 20 percent of all depressive disorders. Unlike unipolar depression, bipolar depression affects men and women about equally.

The symptoms of bipolar disorder vary greatly from person to person. Generally speaking, the depressive symptoms are similar to those we've already described—sadness, low energy, somatic complaints such as headache and stomachache, and poor self-esteem. During a manic phase, the mood is different: People report feeling elated, stronger and smarter than ever, and very passionate about life and their part in it. The "highs" of mania can be quite dangerous, with people taking more physical, sexual, and emotional risks than usual. However, some people with bipolar disorder experience "hypomania," a less intense mood of well-being and confidence that does not significantly interfere with daily life.

According to the *DSM-IV*, a diagnosis of a manic episode is based on the following criteria:

▼ A distinct period of an abnormally and persistently elevated, expansive, or irritable mood that lasts at least one week or requires hospitalization.
▼ During this period, at least three of the following symptoms (four if the only change in mood is increased irritability) have occurred to a significant degree:
    inflated self-esteem or grandiosity
    decreased need for sleep (e.g., feeling rested after three hours of sleep)
    more talkative than usual or feelings of pressure to keep talking
    disconnected and racing thoughts
    distractibility

increase in goal-directed activity (socially, sexually, at work or school) or physical and mental restlessness or agitation

excessive involvement in pleasurable activities that are likely to lead to painful consequences, such as buying sprees or sexual indiscretions

▼ Marked impairment in one's ability to work or engage in usual social activities or relationships, or a need for hospitalization to prevent harm to oneself or others.

▼ The episode is not due to the direct effects of a medication, illicit drug, or medical condition.

The cycles of mania and depression can vary greatly. Initially, the period between episodes of depression, mania, and normal mood are relatively short. In time, the interval between emotional extremes may grow longer. About 5 to 15 percent of those with bipolar disorder experience "rapid cycling," which includes four or more manic or depressive episodes in a year, each lasting at least 24 hours and ending with a switch to the opposite psychological state. In ultrarapid cycling, episodes of depression, mania, or hypomania may last only 24 hours. Like unipolar depression, bipolar disorder may follow a seasonal pattern, with individuals sinking into depression at regular times each year, then swinging into a manic phase at the start of the next season.

Major depression, dysthymia, seasonal affective disorder, premenstrual dysphoric disorder, postpartum depression, bipolar disorder—the range of causes, symptoms, and courses of mood disorders reflects the highly complex nature of brain chemistry as it affects general health, personality, and social functioning. As complicated as depression can be, however, it isn't always the only mental problem involved.

WHEN DEPRESSION IS NOT ALONE

Do you feel panicky and anxious? Do painful memories of a past trauma sometimes overwhelm you? And do these feelings coexist with persistent depressive symptoms? According to the Depression Guideline Panel, a group of mental health experts assembled by the U.S. Department of Health and Human Services, more than 43 percent of people with major depressive disorder have histories of one or more "nonmood" psychiatric disorders. It is important that therapists recognize and then treat all concurrent psychological problems; failing to address one will almost always lead to relapse and further complications.

The most common comorbid conditions with depression (conditions that occur at the same time as depression) include drug and alcohol addiction, anxiety and panic disorders, eating disorder, and posttraumatic stress disorder. We discuss each of these conditions below.

Alcohol and Drug Addiction

Almost any chemical substance we ingest—from illegal drugs like cocaine and marijuana, to liquor, to prescription drugs—may affect our brain's chemistry and thus our moods. Like depression, addiction appears to have a genetic connection, with children of addicted adults more likely to develop an addiction than those without a family history. Also like depression, addiction appears to involve a disruption of brain chemicals combined with psychological and psychosocial factors.

Here, as in many of the medical conditions that mask or trigger depression, the line between cause and effect is a thin and wavering one. Some researchers believe that many substance abusers first start drinking or using drugs to "self-medicate," to relieve painful mood symptoms. If these people also have a vulnerability for addiction, the use of substances to alleviate mood can become a vicious cycle: The physical, social, and psychological problems caused by substance abuse only bring addicts further down, feeling even more useless, hopeless, and sad—and thus needing more alcohol, cocaine, or other substances to lift them up.

Addiction and alcoholism are complicated disorders, with complex causes, courses, and treatment options, and it goes far beyond the scope of this book to cover these problems in any depth. Suffice it to say, it is extremely important that you give your therapist a complete and honest rundown of your use (or abuse) of alcohol or drugs. Only then can he or she make an accurate diagnosis and devise an effective treatment plan that works to address all of your problems.

Anxiety Disorders

The term "anxiety disorders" is used to describe several different types of symptoms, including panic attacks (sudden, inexplicable terror), inordinate fears of certain objects or activities (phobias), or chronic distress and general diffuse feelings of fear (generalized anxiety disorder). According to the National Comorbidity Survey, as many as 25 percent of adult Americans may experience an anxiety disorder over the course of a lifetime. Women are more than twice as likely as men to experience panic attacks and generalized anxiety disorder, especially in combination with depression.

The correlation between depression and anxiety disorders is high. Panic disorders now appear to be present in about 10 to 20 percent of men and women with major depression, and more than 30 percent of depressed people also suffer symptoms of general anxiety disorder. Again, the line between the two is unclear. In some cases, the disruption of brain chemistry involved in depression appears to trigger the panic and anxiety attacks. In others, the stress of dealing with panic and anxiety can so demoralize, isolate, and stigmatize its sufferers, they may well become depressed.

It is extremely important for concurrent anxiety and depression to be treated. The combination can trigger deeper and longer depressions, and considerably raise the risk of suicide. Treatment of a comorbid anxiety disorder and depression frequently involves using a combination of medications and psychotherapeutic approaches. We'll explore these issues in more depth later in the book.

Eating Disorders

"Which is the chicken and which is the egg?" Marilyn considers. "I've always wondered which came first in my life, my depression or my bulimia. Was I so depressed about myself that throwing up seemed a logical solution, or was the secret that I was bulimic bringing me down? Or did the bulimia alter my brain chemistry to make me depressed? I don't know."

Marilyn is not alone in her situation. Studies suggest that between 50 and 75 percent of eating-disorder patients (most of whom are women) suffer from some sort of major depression over their lifetime. Anorexia nervosa affects approximately 0.5 to 1 percent of young women in their late teens and early twenties. It appears to be increasing in incidence in older women and in men. Ninety percent of anorexics are women. The disorder involves a distortion of body image that leads to self-starvation.

Although hungry and with an abnormal obsession with food, those with anorexia force themselves not to eat. Neither weight loss nor dieting decreases their fear of fatness, nor does any amount of logical reasoning break the destructive pattern of denying food, weighing themselves, and fearing food.

Bulimia, which usually includes binging (eating more than 4,000 calories in an hour) and vomiting (or purging), is even more common among young women. According to the *DSM-IV*, 1 to 3 percent of adolescent and young adult women develop bulimia. Risk factors include a previous history of anorexia and a family history of major depression.

Like depression, eating disorders—including obesity, compulsive eating, and binge eating, in addition to anorexia and bulimia—involve a disruption of brain chemistry as well as psychosocial stresses. Serotonin, one of the main neurotransmitters associated with depression, is also implicated in most cases of eating disorders. As we'll discuss in chapter 3, consuming carbohydrates helps to boost serotonin levels, which may help lift mood and return some balance to one's self-perception.

Treatment of eating disorders usually involves a combination of medication (usually antidepressants) and psychotherapy. Again, as is true for all comorbid conditions, it is important for you to discuss any eating-related problems with your doctor or therapist at the same time that you address your depression.

Posttraumatic Stress Disorder

"The memories of my grandfather touching me didn't even enter my conscious until I was nearly forty," explains

Peri. "I'd already been treated once for depression when my first marriage ended when I was twenty-eight, but I didn't remember anything about the abuse until I started getting involved in a new relationship last year. Now I'm working on a whole bunch of issues I never knew I had."

Peri's experience is shared by millions of Americans. The lifetime prevalence of posttraumatic stress disorder (PTSD)—the term applied to any persistent and distressing response to a disturbing, threatening event—is estimated to be about 5 to 14 percent. Most men who develop PTSD do so after taking part in military combat. Most women develop PTSD as a result of being raped, sexually abused, or physically assaulted in some other way. Symptoms of PTSD include vivid nightmares, recurrent or intrusive thoughts about the event (flashbacks), anger, irritability, feelings of emotional numbness and detachment from others, difficulty concentrating, and depression. Treatment usually involves both antidepressant medication and psychotherapy.

As you can see, your mental, emotional, and physical lives are intimately intertwined, and what affects one part of the body or mind is likely to have widespread effects. Now it's time to gain a deeper understanding of what actually happens, in the brain and throughout the body, when a depressive illness takes hold. In chapter 3, we'll show you what scientists know about the biology and pathology of depression.

IMPORTANT QUESTIONS AND ANSWERS ABOUT CHAPTER 2

Q. My sister has no energy, she's lost interest in everything, and has become something of a hypochondriac, always complaining of aches and pains and headaches. I think she's depressed but she denies it. Is it possible to be depressed and not know it?

A. Not only is it possible, but it's quite common. Remember, there are any number of reasons why people tend to deny that their problems are emotional in nature: fear of rejection, shame, and guilt are just a few. And because so many physical illnesses cause symptoms similar to those of depression, your sister may feel that it's easier and/or "more normal" to attribute her problems to a lingering cold or to "just feeling rundown" than to seek psychological help. Discuss your concerns with her as gently and compassionately as you can, and encourage her to see her doctor for a check-up and evaluation if she continues to feel poorly.

Q. I've been feeling low and unhappy for a while now and so made an appointment with a therapist a friend recommended. Should this therapist perform any medical tests on me before making a diagnosis?

A. That depends on several factors, including your symptoms, the therapist's qualifications (is he or she a medical doctor?), and when you last had a complete physical. Certainly, if you haven't had a check-up within a year or so, or have any other reason to suspect that your problems might be physical in origin, see your primary physician as soon as you can. If you see a therapist who is a medical doctor, he or she may recommend laboratory tests (perhaps to test your thyroid function, for instance) should your symptoms warrant it.

Q. I just had a baby who keeps me awake all night. I've hardly had any sleep in a month. Could that be why I feel so sad and desperate all the time, or could I be suffering from postpartum depression?

A. As we'll discuss in chapter 3, there exists an important link between your body's internal clock (the one that regulates your sleeping and eating patterns) and your emotional life. In a branch of medicine called *chronobiology*, scientists study these rhythms and patterns to see how they affect our general health. Of course, whether or not your lack of sleep combined with other physical or emotional factors have triggered a full-blown postpartum depression or if you'll quickly and naturally recover once your baby starts to sleep through the night is a matter for you and your doctor to discuss at length.

3

▼

THE BIOLOGY AND PATHOLOGY OF DEPRESSION

Who, what, why, where, when, and how? These are the six questions every investigative journalist is trained to ask in order to track down the salient facts of a news story. In looking at depression, we've tried to do the same thing. So far, we know something about the "who" of depression. Although anyone can become depressed, more women than men, more people in their early twenties to mid-forties than in other age groups, and more people with a family history of depression than those without a genetic connection tend to become depressed.

We've also explored the "what" of depression: its symptoms and course, as well as the diseases that it can trigger, mask, and/or resemble. We've discussed some of what science knows about the "why" of depression: the factors in someone's genetic makeup and psychosocial history that leave her vulnerable to depression's biochemical changes. In chapter 4, we'll explore more about the "when" of depression: at what points in a woman's life she is more likely to become depressed.

In this chapter, we'll show you the "where" of depression: the places in the brain and body the disorder takes hold. We'll also talk about the "how" of depression: how physiologic and biochemical changes produce symptoms of sadness, emptiness, discomfort, and in rare cases, such hopelessness that suicide seems the only release. We do so by exploring three relatively new branches of medicine currently forging a new understanding of health and healing. Although their names may be complex, and their concepts unfamiliar to you, they represent science's latest and best efforts to understand how the human brain and body do their incredible work.

A branch of medicine known as *biopsychiatry* or *neurobiology* (and its applied sector, psychopharmacology) explores how brain chemistry affects mood and emotions and vice versa. *Psychoneuroimmunology* relates psychology (the study of behavior, emotions, and the mind), neurology (the study of the nervous system), and immunology (the study of the study of the immune system, the disease-fighting cells of the body). A branch of medicine known as *chronobiology* studies the importance of natural body rhythms to overall mental and physical health.

Later in the chapter, we'll show you how much these unofficial offshoots of modern medicine contribute to our current understanding of depression and other mental disorders. In the meantime, let's take a look at what science knows about where in the body our emotions and moods live. You may find this exploration both interesting and helpful in assessing your own mental health issues, as Beth discovered.

"All my life I'd felt weak somehow, morally and spiritually. When I first got help, I didn't bother to look at the biology of my disease. I just took the medication and, even though it made me feel better, I somehow still felt like I wasn't strong enough to do it on my own. Finally, I read a book about depression that really explained what was going on in my brain. And I realized that although I'd made lots of mistakes because I was depressed, the depression itself wasn't my fault. It wasn't because I was weak. This knowledge kind of lifted the blanket of guilt that had been holding me back even more. I know depression, for me, is a lifelong problem, but now I know it's a physical illness, like diabetes or something, rather than a moral failing."

THE BRAIN AND EMOTION

Medical researchers have dubbed the brain "medicine's last frontier" and the 1990s the "Decade of the Brain." Indeed, scientists estimate that they've learned a full 95 percent of what they know about brain anatomy and physiology during the last decade alone. What they've discovered is that the "mind" (thoughts, emotions, moods, and memories) and the "brain" (tissues, chemicals, and nerve cells) are not separate entities but instead intimately intertwined. Mental experiences affect the way the brain functions, and brain processes affect the way we think, feel, and behave. This understanding has led to more effective treatment for mental disorders, since it recognizes both their biological and psychological aspects.

The human brain and nervous system form a vast communications network, one larger and more complex than the long distance companies that span the globe. Every emotion we feel, action we take, and physiologic function we undergo is processed through the brain and the nerve fibers that extend down the spinal cord and throughout the body.

The brain itself is divided into several large regions, each of which is responsible for certain activities. The brain stem, a primitive structure at the base of the skull, controls basic physiological functions such as heart rate and respiration. The cerebral cortex is the largest and most highly developed portion of the brain. Divided into four lobes, the cortex is the center of the brain's higher powers where the activities we define as "thinking"— thought, perception, memory, and communication—take place.

On top of the brain stem and buried under the cortex is another set of structures called the *limbic system.* Scientists believe this highly complex, and still largely unmapped, region is "home base" to our emotions. It receives and regulates emotional information and helps to govern sexual desire, appetite, and stress. Three main centers of the limbic system are the thalamus-hypothalamus, the hippocampus, and the amygdala. The thalamus-hypothalamus forms a kind of "brain within the brain," regulating a variety of human processes, including appetite, thirst, sleep, and certain aspects of mood and behavior. The hippocampus and amygdala help to create memory as well as to gauge emotions.

Thanks to the remarkable advances made in medical technology, scientists have been able to trace how the limbic system registers emotion, and then produces emotional reactions in cooperation with other parts of the brain and body. Studies performed at the National Institute of Mental Health and published in the March 1995 issue of the *American Journal of Psychiatry* hint at the complexity of this process. These experiments show, for instance, that emotional opposites like happiness and sadness involve quite independent patterns of activity. When we feel happy, activity in the region of the cerebral cortex responsible for forethought and planning decreases dramatically, as does activity in the amygdala. When we're unhappy, on the other hand, the amygdala and another part of the cortex become more active.

This division of labor within the brain may be why we're able to experience a seemingly contradictory feeling like "bittersweetness." At our child's high school graduation, for instance, we can feel both happy to see our child pass a remarkable milestone and also sad at the loss of his childhood and the relentless passage of time.

When it comes to depression, the studies showed something else quite interesting. It seems that the same area of the brain—the left prefrontal cortex—appears to be involved in both depression and ordinary sadness, but in different ways. It becomes more active during ordinary sadness, but almost completely shuts down with depression. That might explain the emptiness and numbness many depressed people report. Furthermore, it also appears that men and women might process sadness very differently. In women, sadness causes much more activity in the brain than it does in men, a clue perhaps to how and why women tend to experience periods of more profound sadness than men—and suffer twice the rate of depression.

Sadness, joy, dread, regret, wistfulness, anticipation, awe . . . the extraordinary variety, subtlety, and depth of human emotion is perhaps our most treasured quality, and our ability to experience emotion our most precious gift. It is also a sign of health and vitality. When we are well, we have a full complement of emotions available to us. While each of us has our own unique personality and range of moods, being healthy means being able to experience joy as well as sadness, anger as well as passivity, contentedness as well as frustration. For this to occur, brain cells must be able to communicate with one another, to send messages from one cell to the next, and from one center of brain activity to the other.

Mapping the Synapse

How are these messages sent and received? Let's say you read about a grisly murder in the newspaper. How does the information pass through the parts of the brain that recognize letters and comprehend words, and then go on to structures in the limbic system that trigger emotions like anger and fear? To answer these questions, scientists study not only the anatomy of the brain—its larger structures and organization—but also the biochemical processes that take place among the tiniest cells of the nervous system.

Each nerve cell, or neuron, contains three important parts: the central body, the dendrites, and the axon. Messages from other nerve cells enter the cell body through the dendrites, branchlike projections extending from the cell body. Once the central cell body processes the messages, it can then pass on the information to its neighboring neuron through a cablelike fiber called the axon. In speeds faster than you can imagine, information about every aspect of human physiology, emotion, and thought zips through the body from one neuron to another in precisely this manner.

But there's a hitch: The axon of one neuron does not attach directly to its neighboring nerve cell. Instead, a tiny gap separates the terminal of one axon from the dendrites of the neuron with which it seeks to communicate. This gap is called a synapse. For a message to make it across a synapse, it requires the help of neurotransmitters, chemicals stored in packets at the end of each nerve cell. When a cell is ready to send a message, its axon releases a certain amount and type of neurotransmitter. This chemical then diffuses across the synapse to bind to special molecules, called receptors, that sit on the surface of the dendrites of the adjacent nerve cell.

When a neurotransmitter couples to a receptor, it is like a key fitting into a starter that triggers a biochemical process in that neuron. The receptor molecules link up with other molecules in the cell body, completing the transmission of the message. Once this occurs, whatever amount of neurotransmitter remains in the synapse is either destroyed or, in a process called "reuptake," sucked back into the nerve cell that released it.

Scientists have named forty to fifty neurotransmitters and believe at least fifty more are yet to be identified. Each must be present in sufficient amounts for the brain and nervous system to function properly. When too much or too little neurotransmitter exists, or if the cells are unable to use the chemicals properly, mental and physical disturbances may occur. Indeed, biochemical balance appears to be an important key to mental health.

THE BODY AS CHEMISTRY LAB

"Behind every crooked thought there lies a crooked molecule," the late neuroscientist Ralph Gerard once wrote. The branch of medicine called neurobiology explores that very notion by attempting to identify, and then to resolve, the chemical imbalances that are often at the heart of mental disorders like depression.

As discussed, in most cases of mental illness, chemicals called neurotransmitters—substances that allow nerve cells to communicate with each other—are not present in the right amounts or are not used efficiently. An imbalance of three neurotransmitters—serotonin, dopamine, and nor-epinephrine—appears to be involved in most cases of depression. These same chemical imbalances also occur in people who suffer from anxiety, eating disorders, obsessive-compulsive disorder, and several other psychological disturbances.

When it comes to depression, scientists have identified serotonin as the most common and likely culprit. With the most extensive network of any neurotransmitter, serotonin influences a wide range of brain activities, including mood, behavior, movement, pain, sexual activity, appetite, hormone secretion, and heart rate. People with depression have been found to have lower amounts than usual of serotonin in the brain, as have people suffering from bulimia. As you'll see in chapter 5, drugs that help more serotonin to remain available in the synapse—called SSRIs or selective serotonin reuptake inhibitors—are often very successful in alleviating depression.

Another important neurotransmitter is dopamine, which follows two main pathways in the brain. One pathway connects to a portion of the brain called the corpus striatum, which controls movement. When this pathway malfunctions, as it does in diseases such as Parkinson's disease and Huntington's chorea, problems with muscle control arise. The ocher dopamine pathway extends into the limbic system. When dopamine does not exist in proper amounts or is unable to reach organs of the limbic system, emotional problems such as depression may occur.

Norepinephrine is the third neurotransmitter thought to be involved in depression. Lower than normal amounts of this neurotransmitter have been measured in people who are depressed, as well as in people suffering with the eating disorder called anorexia. Scientists have found a few different medications that help restore proper norepinephrine levels in the brain.

Like serotonin, norepinephrine molecules contain only one of a certain kind of protein, called an amine, so it is classified as a monoamine. One class of drugs developed to help alleviate depression concentrates on preventing a substance called monoamine oxidase from breaking down monoamines like norepinephrine and serotonin. When medication (called monoamine oxidase inhibitors or MAOIs) stops the action of this substance, more norepinephrine and serotonin are available to nerve cells, allowing cells to send and receive the right signals. Tricyclic antidepressants, discussed in chapter 5, also work on restoring norepinephrine (as well as serotonin) activity.

As technology continues to improve, scientists will learn even more about these neurotransmitters and how they affect emotion, thought, and behavior. In the meantime, they've already discovered that neurotransmitters do not work alone in transmitting messages, but instead cooperate directly with another system of the body: the endocrine system, which produces chemicals called hormones.

The Endocrine Connection

What lets your brain "know" that your stomach is empty and makes you feel hungry? What causes you to feel sleepy at night? How does your uterus know when it's time to expel an unfertilized egg? Why does your heart beat faster when something frightens or excites you?

The answer to all of these questions is the same: Hormones, chemicals produced by the glands of the endocrine system, trigger the onset or termination of these and other actions and reactions. They work with neurotransmitters as messengers, sending information and instructions to organs and cells throughout the body. In fact, several chemicals are both neurotransmitters and hormones, depending upon where they work and what messages they are meant to transmit. Norepinephrine, for instance, acts as a neurotransmitter in the brain, while it performs as a hormone on the heart and blood vessels during times of stress.

When it comes to depression, three areas of the endocrine system appear to be directly involved. As you may remember from chapter 2, the thyroid gland produces hormones that affect our emotions, as well as regulate our metabolism. When the thyroid becomes hyperactive, it may produce symptoms that resemble mania—hyperactivity, overexcitement, loss of appetite, and insomnia, among others. When it becomes underactive, symptoms associated with major depression—excessive sleepiness, lethargy, and sadness—may occur.

In addition, women have powerful sex hormones that surge and ebb on a cyclical basis. Since the endocrine system works as a unit, with the level of one hormone influencing the levels of all others, this cycle has a profound effect on far more than our reproductive lives. The mood swings and depression many women feel just before or during their periods is one example of the impact sex hormones have on our mental health; the anxiety and sadness of postpartum depression is another.

A third important endocrine connection to depression is called the HPA axis because it involves the hypothalamus, pituitary, and adrenal glands. The HPA axis is involved in the regulation of *cortisol*, a steroid hormone secreted during prolonged stress as well as at regular intervals throughout the day. Whenever the brain senses danger or difficulty, it responds by sending chemical signals that prepare the body to either fight or flee the impending situation. Called the "fight or flight" response, this reaction involves the release of cortisol from the adrenal glands. Cortisol then converts norepinephrine into epinephrine, or adrenalin, which gets your heart pumping harder, your muscles tensed for action, your sweat glands open, and your mind more alert.

Scientists studying depression discovered that a large percentage of seriously depressed people have a much higher level of cortisol in their bloodstreams than normal. Strangely enough, although depression usually causes a *decrease* in feelings of agitation and activity (just the sort of biological state cortisol triggers), cortisol levels in depressed people are even higher than in people with disorders more commonly associated with extreme stress, like anxiety and psychosis.

What causes cortisol levels to be so high in depression is still under investigation. As you'll see later in the chapter when we talk about chronobiology, cortisol is one of the many hormones the body produces on a relatively automatic, time-released basis. Some researchers believe that our internal rhythms of hormone production may become irregular and out-of-sync, causing a host of physiological and emotional symptoms. Another theory postulates that depression somehow causes the HPA axis to malfunction so that the body is unable to stop cortisol production after stress has passed. Suffering from prolonged stress, then, is a triggering factor for depression in many individuals.

EMOTION IS EVERYWHERE

From across a crowded room, you see the man you love. He turns and smiles. Your heart races, your palms sweat, your breathing quickens. These very physical reactions to an emotional encounter show in a clear and direct way that body and mind are not at all separate, but are one and the same. Your emotions are directly linked to your physical self.

It should come as no surprise, then, that the way you think and feel about yourself and your life might have an impact on your physical health. Think how often you've heard about one or more of these situations: A wife falls ill and passes away within just a few months of her husband's death. A businesswoman working overtime under the stress of an impending deadline develops a head cold she just can't shake. A grandmother seems to will herself to live just long enough to see her granddaughter's college graduation. An otherwise secure young woman succumbs to depression as she struggles to control a nagging case of chronic asthma.

A new branch of medicine called *psychoneuroimmunology* presents a remarkable explanation for these seemingly coincidental events: Your nervous system is intimately intertwined with your immune system, the cells of the body that fight disease. The activity of one system directly impacts on the other.

One study conducted at the University of California at Los Angeles involved actors, individuals who by nature and training are able to elicit from themselves strong emotions on cue. As the actors experienced a certain emotion, researchers tested their hormones and blood to see what changes occurred. They found that certain white blood cells—cells important in fighting infection—increased in both number and activity level. This increase occurred no matter what kind of emotion, positive or negative, the actors evoked.

At first glance, it might seem that having an emotional crisis could actually work to fight disease since it triggers the immune system to take action. But researchers postulate that the immune system becomes overworked if constantly stimulated, eventually losing its effectiveness and leaving the body open to disease. This would explain why illness tends to occur during, or immediately following, periods of stress. It would also show another link between depression and many physical illnesses. Why it is, according to recent studies, that severely depressed heart attack patients are about five times as likely to die within six months of leaving the hospital as patients who aren't depressed?

Exactly how thoughts and emotions act on immune system cells is still not fully understood. It appears that the brain is capable of triggering the immune system to perform in certain ways—the same way that the brain, when it senses fear, can trigger the heart to beat faster. Another connection between the brain and immune system involves chemicals called neuropeptides. Like neurotransmitters, these chemicals were once thought to exist only in the brain, but have since been found throughout the body. According to current theory, these chemicals may be the physical representations of emotions. Neuropeptides control, for instance, the opening and closing of blood vessels in the face. When you suddenly feel embarrassed, these chemicals are responsible for the blush that rushes to your cheeks.

Precisely where does depression fit into the psychoneuroimmunologic picture? That remains to be seen. For now, it is important to understand that calling depression a "mental illness" without recognizing its physical aspects is both arbitrary and ultimately self-defeating. It also behooves us to keep in mind that suffering from depression can leave us more vulnerable to a host of other illnesses as well, both psychiatric (like anxiety disorders or substance abuse) and medical (like heart disease and cancer).

TIMING IS EVERYTHING

Almost everyone living in the modern age has experienced what is familiarly known as "jet lag." You arrive in Paris from Los Angeles after a grueling trip across nine time zones. You feel disoriented, exhausted, even a little queasy and ill. You feel this way for a day or two, until your body catches up with the local environment, until you feel tired when the natives feel tired and feel hungry just as the aroma of *pommes frites* wafts out of bistros at Parisian lunch and dinnertime.

But what would happen if you never adjusted? If your body remained out-of-sync with your environment? What if there are events other than traveling through time zones that upset our body clocks—like a physical illness or an emotional crisis? Many scientists, especially those involved in the study of body rhythms called *chronobiology*, believe that such unintentional disruptions do occur and that they may well be responsible for any number of mental and physical disorders, including depression.

Far more than we realize, our internal and external lives are regulated by rhythms of light and dark, of sleep and wakefulness, of fluctuating body temperature, blood pressure, and hormone secretion. Researchers believe that our rhythms are driven by two different oscillators: One is very consistent and controls body temperature and many hormonal secretions. The other oscillator is more fluid and subject to change, and controls sleep/wake and activity/rest patterns. Chronobiologists think that it is when these two oscillators become desynchronized that illness— mental or physical—may occur.

What sets up these physiological cycles and keeps them on schedule? There are many different "zeitgebers" (as the term is known in German) or "time-keepers" that establish our body clocks. Some zeitgebers are internal, set up and maintained regardless of external factors. (These are the more consistent ones.) Others depend heavily on cues we receive from the outside world: the knowledge we have of time established by clocks and watches (how often have we suddenly felt hungry only when we noticed it's "lunch time"), the smell of coffee brewing in the morning, the sound of traffic picking up during rush hour in the afternoon.

Perhaps the strongest and best known zeitgeber is the sun: The light it brings each morning and takes away at dusk triggers the release or inactivation of certain hormones that trigger our mood and behavior. For example, we don't go to sleep when it's dark only out of habit, or because darkness makes activity more difficult, or even just because we're tired. It's largely because the body produces a hormone called melatonin—also known as "the chemical expression of darkness"—when the eyes tell the brain that it is dark.

Once produced, melatonin then signals to the rest of the body that it is time to rest. When the sun comes up, the body stops producing melatonin, which triggers the release of more action-oriented hormones, such as cortisol. Our body temperature and blood pressure begin to rise, revving the body up for daytime activity. That's why jet lag feels so odd: Our bodies continue to produce "waking" hormones even when its dark, and circulate "sleeping" hormones when it's light until our external and internal zeitgebers have a chance to coordinate with one another.

Chronobiologists have discovered a number of fascinating things about how these rhythms affect our health. Did you know that the length of time you sleep is related more closely to your body temperature and bedtime than how long you've been awake? Experiments show that even after being awake more than twenty hours, people free of time cues slept twice as long when they went to bed when their temperature was at its highest (in early evening) than it was at its lowest (in the early morning). Your senses of hearing, taste, and smell tend to be most acute—strangely enough—in the middle of the night (around 3 A.M.), then fall off during the morning, then rise again to a new high between 5 and 7 P.M., which may be one of the reasons why the evening meal tends to be more sumptuous than breakfast or lunch.

Did you know that heart attacks are more likely to occur in the morning than in the evening? One reason is because more cortisol—the stress-related hormone that causes the heart rate and blood pressure to rise is secreted in larger amounts in the morning hours than later in the day. Asthma attacks are also more likely to take place in the early morning when lung function is at a daily low. Pain tolerance is highest in the afternoon, which is why it might make sense for you to visit the dentist or participate in strenuous activity at this time.

The Rhythms of Depression

Chronobiology also explores the effect rhythms have on our mental health, including their influence on depression and bipolar disorder. It seems logical to assume there's a connection, since so many of the classic somatic symptoms of depression—sleeping difficulties, changes in appetite and eating habits, poor concentration—are related to regular rhythms of life. Some of these rhythms are circadian in nature, which means that they occur in cycles of roughly twenty-four hours. Blood pressure, heart rate, the sleep/wake cycle, appetite, some aspects of sleep itself, and body temperature are just a few examples of circadian rhythms.

Recent studies show that circadian rhythms in depressed people are significantly off-kilter when compared with the daily rhythms of healthy individuals. Normal nighttime increases in melatonin secretion are absent in three out of four depressed people studied; in patients with bipolar disorder, the melatonin rhythm seems completely desynchronized, with more melatonin produced during depressive phases and less during manic periods. One reason for this disruption is that melatonin is derived from the neurotransmitter serotonin, which is also in an imbalanced state in most people with depression and bipolar disorder.

Sleep is what suffers most from the melatonin imbalance, with most depressed people sleeping much more or much less than usual. In addition, the pattern of sleep itself is different. Normally, sleep consists of four stages plus REM (rapid eye movements), the near waking state during which we dream. These stages occur in repeating 90-minute cycles throughout the night, with REM occupying as little as ten minutes per cycle at the beginning of sleep, then increasing in length toward morning. With depression, REM sleep occurs far more quickly after the onset of sleep and diminishes toward morning.

Some chronobiological rhythms are seasonal, although they tend to be more subtle in humans because we are exposed to indoor lighting and heating. Studies show, for instance, that more women conceive during the summer than in the winter in northern countries in which a strong seasonal contrast in light/dark patterns exists. This means that more babies are born in the inviting spring rather than in the dark cold of winter. Both men and women tend to eat about 220 more calories a day in the fall than in any other season and, even though we are eating more food, we feel hungrier at this time. Anthropologists suggest that we eat more during this time because we're unconsciously storing fat for the winter as we did before refrigerators and freezers made food plentiful year-round. (Unfortunately for us, women more than men tend to show the effects of this seasonal appetite fluctuation: We gain more fat and muscle mass during the fall and winter than men do.)

Mental illness also has its seasons. Episodes of depression and bipolar disorder occur much more in fall and winter than they do in spring and summer. This tendency is so pervasive that a category of depression called SAD (seasonal affective disorder) has been created.

As discussed earlier, about ten million Americans suffer with SAD every year, usually in the months from October through April. Because the amount of light to which we are exposed lessens significantly during the winter, scientists believe that people with SAD—most of whom are women—may be particularly sensitive to the concurrent increase in melatonin secretion.

As the science of chronobiology continues to expand, we may all begin to better understand what natural rhythms mean to our mental and physical health. Thanks to the monthly cycle of menstruation, which follows the cycle of the moon, women have always been more attuned to and sensitive to natural rhythms and their biological and psychological imperatives. When these rhythms become desynchronized for any reason, we become sad, unfocused, out-of-sorts, ill. Most of us are able to restore balance with medication, with therapy, or through the physiological changes that come with the passage of time. Others, however, are not. For them, suicide seems the only way to stop the pain.

WHEN LIVING IS TOO
LARGE A BURDEN

"I just couldn't bear to be alive anymore," Beth remembers. "The pain, the emptiness, the look of pity and fear in my family's eyes. The thought of seeing myself in the mirror one more morning was unbearable to me. There was no hope. Nothing was ahead of me but more pain, more disappointment. So I hoarded some painkillers my husband had left over from an injury and took them all one afternoon. If my sister hadn't come along when she did, I wouldn't be here today."

Beth, who attempted suicide seven years ago at the age of forty-four, has come a long way since then. Although once again in the midst of a depressive episode, she has learned to recognize the danger signs and seek help before the despair and loneliness become too great. Beth is one of the lucky ones—at least 30,000 people (some estimate the number is closer to 75,000) end their own lives every year, and the overwhelming majority of them suffer from depression or other mental disorder.

Suicide is a complex issue. It is not in itself a mental disorder, but is often the final act in a long tragedy of mental illness. The common thread in all suicides is a profound lack of hope that life will get better, that there remains anything in the present or future worth the struggle against overwhelming physical and/or emotional pain.

What brings someone to this point? Without question, depression and suicide often go hand in hand, and recent evidence suggests several similarities between the two problems. Like depression, suicide has a familial component. Relatives of suicides have nearly a ten times higher risk of suicide than those without a family history. Moreover, up to 50 percent of adolescent suicides or suicide attempters have at least one suicidal first-degree relative (parent, child, sibling).

There also appear to be similar brain chemistry imbalances in those who are depressed and those who are suicidal, namely a shortage of the neurotransmitters serotonin and norepinephrine. Research has shown that well over 95 percent of suicides' brains have deficiencies in serotonin and—remarkably—the more violent (and thus definite) means used to kill oneself, the lower the amount of serotonin in the brain. Other factors influencing suicidal behavior are as follows:

Age

Although depression rates begin to slowly rise as children enter puberty, suicide rates absolutely soar. Over the past thirty years, rates for young suicides have risen more than 300 percent, making suicide the second biggest killer of American adolescents after accidents. A 1990 Gallup poll showed the extent of this disturbing trend: More than 15 percent of thirteen- to nineteen-year-olds admitted knowing a teenage suicide and 60 percent admitted knowing a teenage suicide attempter. Some studies of college students indicate that up to 20 percent have made, or have seriously considered making, a suicide attempt during their high school years.

Psychiatrists and sociologists continue to search for a reason why so many of our young people want to die. As we'll discuss in chapter 4, adolescence is a time of overwhelming psychosocial and biological pressure, which can result in prolonged and undermining stress. Hormones are raging at this time as well, disrupting regular body rhythms and setting the stage for chemical imbalances.

Gender

The gender gap for suicide is almost exactly the reverse of the one for depression: Men are three times more likely to take their own lives than women. Elderly men are ten times more likely to take their own lives than elderly women, and the incidence of suicide among teenage boys is twice as high as among girls.

However, while women are about three times as likely to *attempt* suicide than are men, most of these attempts are unsuccessful. One reason is that women usually choose much less violent—and thus more ambivalent— means of ending their lives. Men are far more likely to use a gun or hang themselves, while women tend to overdose on drugs or attempt to suffocate themselves with carbon monoxide or gas. Because these latter methods tend to take longer to succeed and are far less consistent in their effects, women are often saved by an intervening friend or relative.

The highest rates of suicide across the population are among older men: 25 percent of all suicides occur in men over the age of sixty-five. Male rates jump from about 10 in 100,000 for young adolescents, to 25 in 100,000 for young adults, then rise to about 35 in 100,000 for those aged sixty-five to seventy-four, then increase to about 60 in 100,000 in the oldest age group. In contrast, female rates of suicide are about 5 per 100,000 during adolescence, about 20 per 100,000 in middle age, and drop to less than 10 in the oldest groups.

Why woman are more prone to periods of great despondency, but are usually strong enough to resist the temptation to end the pain by ending their lives is a question that may well be unanswerable. It could be that our ties to the earth and to each other are too great to abandon: We give birth, we nurture both our children and our families, and we are the caretakers. We tend to talk more openly about our feelings than men do (at least until recently) and thus are able to give and receive more support. It could also be that something about the richness and energy of our cyclical hormonal lives keeps us alive and willing to face another day, another season.

A topic as compelling as suicide deserves a larger forum than the one provided by this book. In the Resource section, you'll find a list of publications and organizations devoted to the topic. In the meantime, it's important for you to understand—and thus be able to recognize—the risk factors and warning signs of suicide.

The Risks Factors and Warning Signs for Suicide

A constellation of influences—mental disorders, personality traits, genetic vulnerability, medical illness, psychosocial stressors—combine to undermine an individual's strength and will to live. Depression and alcoholism are underlying factors in more than two-thirds of all suicides. Other risk factors for suicide include:

▼ Being a psychiatric patient
▼ Being an adolescent or being over the age of seventy
▼ Suffering from mental or psychiatric disorders including depression and alcoholism
▼ Having a history of prior suicide attempts
▼ Experiencing a recent interpersonal loss, especially in alcoholic individuals
▼ Having feelings of low self-esteem and hopelessness
▼ Having a family history of suicide in the last two generations

The three most common warning signs of suicide include:

▼ Extreme changes in behavior
▼ A previous suicide attempt
▼ Any suicidal threat or statement

How many of the risk factors and warning signs apply to you or someone close to you? It may be a cliché, but it is one worth repeating: The best cure for suicide lies in prevention. If you believe you're at risk of taking your life, reach out for help. Talk to your physician, your therapist, your clergyman, your best friend. Do not try to face the darkness alone.

Who, what, where, why, and how . . . we've looked at each of those areas as they relate to depression. Now, in chapter 4, we will explore the *when* of this widespread disorder, the times in your life when depression is more likely than others to affect you.

IMPORTANT QUESTIONS AND ANSWERS ABOUT CHAPTER 3

Q. Psychoneuroimmunology sounds a lot like the "power of positive thinking." Can the way we feel or think about something really affect our physical health?

A. Scientists have known for decades that our immune system and our nervous system interact. When fighting an infection, for instance, immune cells are able to stimulate the brain to transmit impulses that produce fever. And receptors for many of the chemicals released during the fight-or-flight stress response have been observed on the surface of lymphocytes near the lymph nodes and in the spleen.

The power of feelings to affect the physical body was dramatically demonstrated in a study performed during the 1980s and released in 1989. Dr. David Spiegel, a psychiatrist at Stanford University, divided a group of eighty-six women, all of whom had metastatic (spreading) breast cancer. One group was given standard medical care—surgery, chemotherapy, and radiation. The members of the other group received the same therapy, but were also asked to meet once a week in a group therapy session in which emotions—often dismissed by physicians concentrating on strictly physical aspects of cancer—were expressed, discussed, and confronted.

The immediate effects surprised few people: The women who had the support of fellow cancer patients and a qualified leader reported fewer symptoms of depression, anxiety, and pain than those in the other group. After all, they had more opportunities to express their emotions and find solutions to problems.

What did surprise Dr. Spiegel and other physicians were the long-range effects of support groups. Several years later, Spiegel made a startling discovery: Those who took part in group psychotherapy—and who suffered less from depression and anxiety—had lived twice as long after they entered the study as the group that received only standard medical care.

Indeed, how you feel does have an impact on your physical health, and vice versa. It is important to understand that connection as you learn more about your own case of depression and how it might be affecting your health.

Q. You mentioned melatonin, the hormone related to sleep and the setting of our body clock. Is melatonin related to serotonin? Does it have a role in depression?

A. Melatonin is derived from serotonin, which is itself a derivative of a substance called tryptophan. Tryptophan is an amino acid, one of twenty-two organic compounds that are the basic building blocks of human life. Amino acids act as regulators of vital body activities, such as those that trigger the production of hormones like serotonin, as well as constitute the primary ingredients of muscles, bones, and other tissues.

The human body does not make tryptophan. We obtain it from the diet, specifically in food high in protein. Once digested, tryptophan is first synthesized into serotonin then, through a complex molecular process, serotonin is later converted into melatonin by the pineal gland, an endocrine gland located in the brain.

Melatonin and serotonin are inextricably linked: When melatonin levels drop or rise for any reason, so do serotonin levels, and vice versa. In those people who are depressed, both serotonin and melatonin levels tend to be much lower than usual. In addition, scientists think that when melatonin levels change, it disrupts the internal body clock—the one that organizes and regulates our physiologic, emotional, and intellectual behavior. This disruption may be another important trigger for depression.

Q. When it comes to suicide, is depression the only factor? I wonder because not all teenage suicides I've read about seem depressed. Instead, they seem more fearful about the future or anxious about fitting in.

A. Your impression is correct. Anxiety seems to be involved in more cases of teen suicide than depression. A study conducted in Chicago showed that only about one out of four of about seventy teenage suicides were severely depressed at the time. However, major depression raises the risk of completed suicide—in teenagers and adults—more than thirtyfold, and thus remains the most serious factor influencing suicidal behavior.

4

▼

THROUGH THE LIFE CYCLE

A Woman's Special Risk

On July 1, 1996, model and actress Margaux Hemingway was found dead in her Santa Monica home. She left no suicide note, but most who knew her suspected that she had succumbed to one of the many demons that had haunted her throughout her life. She had struggled with anorexia and bulimia, alcoholism, and a chronic, underlying depression. As the granddaughter of novelist Ernest Hemingway, who shot himself in 1965, she also inherited the twin burdens of fame and tragedy.

Describing an earlier suicide attempt, Ms. Hemingway told a reporter, "I was trying to live life to the fullest. And I thought that I had to drink and . . . my grandfather's books . . . they are all about eating and drinking. And so it runs in the family. Violence and this fascination with death also."

At first glance, the circumstances of Margaux Hemingway's life and death may seem outside the average woman's universe. She was uncommonly beautiful, famous and, for a time at least, leading the life of a glamorous Hollywood superstar. We saw her in movies, on television, and gracing the covers of magazines.

And yet most of us can imagine and relate to the anxieties and fears Ms. Hemingway apparently harbored. Like many others with mental health problems, she had a family history of both depression and suicide, and the self-defeating patterns of behavior that often follow it. At the same time, she strived for independence and success in a world dominated by men, and in a business that tends to treat women as mere commodities. In a culture that worships beauty, she attempted to starve herself to win approval and love, to control the uncontrollable. And in a culture that still worships youth, she entered her forties worrying about where the next stage of life would take her. She was just forty-one when she died.

There are probably very few of us who haven't felt oppressed by these very same concerns. Those of us susceptible may also fall victim to depression as we attempt to face them, as did Margaux Hemingway. "There used to be an expression 'a woman's lot in life,' that I always resented because it seemed to be a self-fulfilling prophecy," 82-year-old Gloria confesses. "But at the same time, I think the burdens of the many roles we have, and the way men have historically looked down on us for doing what really is some of the most crucial work on the planet, is awfully demoralizing. There's nothing worse than being made to feel unimportant or replaceable. I'm glad to see that things are changing for the better, slowly but surely."

THE TWENTY-FIRST-CENTURY
WOMAN

In many ways, there has never been a better time to be a woman growing older in America. Although we still earn less than men for the same work, our wages have steadily increased during the past few decades while those for men have stayed the same or decreased. The glass ceiling still exists, but it exists on a higher floor in the corporate and professional worlds. Women are still the victims of the majority of domestic and sexual abuse, but we no longer expect to suffer alone or in silence. Every state in the nation offers help in the form of support groups, shelters, and stiffer penalties against offenders. And although women and their children represent the largest proportion by far of poor people in America, women also make up more than 50 percent of the population in law schools and medical schools.

Even more important, we now live longer—life expectancy for the average American woman is about seventy-five years—and in better health than ever before. With this extended life cycle comes exciting challenges for continued growth and change, but also new anxieties about how, or even if, we'll be able to meet those challenges.

In 1975, journalist Gail Sheehy wrote the groundbreaking book *Passages*, in which she chronicled the stages of life, decade by decade, of men and women living in the 1970s. Each stage had pretty clear-cut expectations for women: In your twenties, you married and had children. In your thirties, you took care of those children, your husband, and, often, your aging parents and in-laws. In your forties, you began to wind down or, if you faced divorce, struggled to find your place in an uncomfortable new world. By the time you hit your fifties and sixties, you felt old and you *were* old in the eyes of the increasingly young population growing up around you. At seventy, your life was fundamentally over.

Fortunately, more than two decades of social, political, and medical progress have considerably altered those expectations. In her 1995 bestseller, *New Passages*, Ms. Sheehy describes a completely new set of stages beginning with an adolescence that lasts until almost our thirties and a whole second adulthood we embark upon in our mid-fifties. Within those stages, there is remarkable flexibility about what roles to play and when to play them, at least for well-educated women. A grandmother can go back to college without causing too much of a stir, a mother who works outside the home is the rule rather than the exception, and a fifty-year-old woman who decides never to marry is no longer referred to as an "old maid."

Even circumstances that were once considered biologically restricted by time have been loosened: More women are waiting until their early to mid-forties to have a child, for example, when just a couple of decades ago it was odd to see a new mother over the age of thirty-five. Sex after eighty has come out of the closet, so to speak, and has been encouraged by physicians, explored in magazine articles, and practiced by increasing numbers of less and less inhibited elders.

With all of these choices and options, why do women still become depressed in record numbers? Part of the reason, of course, is biological. After all, a chemical imbalance can occur no matter what your circumstances, especially if you're genetically vulnerable, and the hormonal life of the average woman offers many opportunities for disruption.

Furthermore, while it may seem that we have more choices than ever before, just the opposite may be true— or at least feel that way. It's not just *possible* to have a career and be a wife and mother, it is for most women absolutely *necessary* to do so. Once upon a time, if you reached the age of, say, thirty-five without having a child, no one expected that you ever would. Now the question remains open for another ten years, and many women feel a nagging pressure from within and without to keep that option open. Knowing that a healthy and active sex life is possible throughout your life is indeed liberating, but it may also be intimidating. It means you have to stay feeling—and looking—sexually attractive forever, no easy task in a society that stubbornly clings to the concept of youth equals beauty.

Identifying Your Risks

The truth is that life for the average American woman is still fraught with economic, social, and biological challenges. In addition, there are several personal factors that might increase your own chances of falling victim to depression at some point during your life. See how you relate to these issues.

Your Self-esteem

Self-esteem is a much-touted but rather nebulous term. After all, the way you feel about yourself and your place in the world is highly subjective and very changeable. Nevertheless, the overall value you place on your intelligence, competence, and sociability may well have an impact on your emotional and physical health.

Do you often feel that society in general or the people in your life in particular do not take you seriously? Do you think the role you play in your family and/or community is unimportant? Do you consider physical attractiveness to be a primary measure of your self-worth, and thus feel insecure because you don't measure up to the impossible standards set by the media?

If so, you're not alone. Although the tide may be turning when it comes to the way society views women and the roles we play, centuries of being treated as second-class citizens in a male-dominated world have taken their toll. You've probably had to fight for people to consider your opinions and life choices of equal merit to those of your male peers. That's quite a burden, one that adds a great deal of stress—constant and pervasive—to the universal struggle both men and women wage to define themselves and their roles in society.

Quite apart from these historical and social factors, your level of self-esteem as an adult depends a great deal on how much comfort, support, and encouragement you received from your parents during your childhood. If they were there to clap when you took your first step, to back you up when you felt slighted, and to help you focus on your strengths rather than your weaknesses, chances are better that you grew up to be a strong and centered woman. If not, then you may be more vulnerable to feelings of low self-esteem, and thus to depression. That's why children of alcoholics run a higher risk of developing depression; their parents' addiction and related behaviors often prevent them from receiving the kind of support necessary for healthy development during their formative years.

Your Personal Coping Style

Do you meet new challenges with anticipation and optimism, or apprehension and negativity? When confronting a problem, do you tend to brood about it for a long time, or quickly take action to either resolve it or distract yourself? If you're like most women, you probably spend a lot of time hashing out your problems with friends and dwelling on them during your quiet moments alone. Unfortunately, this tendency may increase your risk for depression.

In fact, one of the reasons psychologists think that men are less likely to become depressed is that men tend to involve themselves in activities, like sports and work, that both divert them and give them a sense of mastery and control. Most women, on the other hand, do not feel as powerful or as in control of their environment, and thus may be more passive and introspective. Whether or not we're born with these gender differences in coping styles or are socialized to behave this way remains a question for anthropologists, neurobiologists, and psychologists to answer. In any case, you might want to consider the way you cope with challenges when assessing your risk for depression.

Ask yourself, too, how you usually cope with changes that occur in your life, either positive or negative. If you have trouble adapting when something alters your circumstances, then you may suffer from increased stress. As you may remember from chapter 3, too much stress may well upset the delicate balance of neurotransmitters in the brain, and thus leave you more susceptible to depression. Although we tend to think of interpersonal loss—the breakup of a marriage, the death of a loved one, an estrangement from one's children or parents—as the likely trigger for most cases of depression, any sudden change in circumstances may cause even more stress. The loss of a job or of financial security, relocating to a different part of the country, an impending emotionally or logistically complicated event—any of these situations can upset your internal balance.

Your Hormonal Makeup and Physiology

From the moment you hit puberty, your physical and emotional life hinges to a great degree on the level and action of hormones—the chemicals that transmit messages about mood, behavior, and function to the organs of the body. In chapter 3, we discussed how hormones work, and how an imbalance or malfunction of these chemicals might influence the development of depression. Later in this chapter, you'll learn more about depression related to premenstrual syndrome—an explicit example of the way hormones can affect mental health.

In addition, the fact that you're female and capable of giving birth brings up several emotional issues: Should you have a child? If so, when? Will you find a man you respect and love enough to share the responsibility? Are you physically capable of bearing a child? What happens to your heart and soul if you're not, or if you suffer a miscarriage? How will society look at you—and how will you feel about yourself—if you decide not to have a child? What if your biological clock runs down before you meet the right man or feel you're ready to have a child on your own?

Questions about motherhood may or may not be crucial to you. You may have become a mother already with relative ease. Or you may have decided long ago—and with confidence—that motherhood was not for you. For a majority of women, though, these issues become a source of stress and anxiety. Coupled with the hormonal changes that occur with menstruation, pregnancy, and birth, this anxiety may trigger depression.

Your Social and Economic Circumstances

You've probably heard the expression "Life is what you make it" and though it sounds a bit trite, to some degree it's also true: Your attitude toward life and the challenges you face can matter more than any one hardship. On the other hand, if you feel trapped by poverty, live in an abusive household, have a chronic medical condition, or have a history of being sexually abused, then the burdens you bear may well tip the scales against your physical and emotional well-being. In fact, most cases of depression are not triggered by the dip in self-esteem or disappointment that come from breaking up with a boyfriend or even the death of a loved one. The loss of a job and financial and personal security that goes with it is often a more devastating source of stress.

How many of these concerns relate to you? Are there aspects about your coping style, personality, or economic circumstances that might make you more susceptible to depression? Do you see how the way you think about yourself or deal with problems might allow depression to get a toehold in your life? These questions are just the sort that psychotherapists are trained to help you work through, while medication can help restore any chemical imbalances that might otherwise undermine your progress. (We discuss the benefits of medication and therapy in more detail in chapters 5, 6, and 7.)

THE TIMES OF YOUR LIFE

In the meantime, it may be helpful to look at the times in your life when depression is more likely to strike than others. In very general terms, a woman's life can be divided into five stages, each with its own set of biological and psychological challenges and risks for depression.

The first section, *Coming into Your Own*, describes the first difficult transition between adolescence and young adulthood, when a woman is most likely to experience premenstrual syndrome for the first time as well as confront an eating disorder. *The Search for a Place in the World* explores what happens to many women after they leave school and begin to realize the challenges of truly being on their own for the first time. *The Tentative Thirties* covers the decade when more and more women choose to make their most crucial decisions about career, marriage, and motherhood. *Consolidating in the Forties* details the decade in which most women begin to assess where life has taken them so far, and what their next step should be. *Forging the Passage* takes place between the ages of fifty and about sixty-five, and includes both menopause and, for most, the transition from working woman (or wife to a working man) and retirement. Finally, there is the stage we call *Heading into Late Life*, which stretches from the late sixties into the eighties, nineties, and beyond. During this period, women tend to encounter grief more often, with friends and siblings succumbing to illness. We often become primary caregivers to our ailing husbands. We become ill ourselves and, eventually, face our own mortality.

Keep in mind that the age at which these milestones occur varies greatly from individual to individual. You may sail through your teens and twenties without a hitch, but succumb to your first bout of depression when a chronic illness like rheumatoid arthritis takes hold in your late thirties. You may have your first child at forty-three and thus still be grappling with the frustrations of early parenthood while your peers are looking toward early retirement. Your first encounter with depression related to premenstrual syndrome might not occur until you're in your late forties, when hormonal changes related to pre-menopause disrupt your chemical balance. That's why you may find it best to read about each of these stages of life, no matter what your age now.

Coming into Your Own

According to information Gail Sheehy gathered for her book *New Passages*, it takes longer to become an adult today than ever before. Adolescence used to span from the time girls got their first periods—usually at twelve or thirteen—until about the age of twenty-one, when they got a job, left college, got married, and/or embarked upon a career. Today, however, girls enter puberty as young as nine or ten and often delay decisions about work and marriage until well into their twenties or later.

A time of great emotional and physical turmoil, adolescence is the period during which a girl strives to separate from her parents, establish her own identity, attain a measure of comfort with her sexuality, and develop an idea of what kind of life she'd like to lead. With all of these challenges converging at once, it's no wonder that many teens suffer depression and anxiety as they attempt to adapt and progress through this rocky period. Unfortunately, it doesn't appear that the extension of adolescence from about eight to ten years to fifteen to twenty years has alleviated any of the angst that tends to accompany these changes. In fact, if suicide rates are any indication, the transition from childhood to maturity is more fraught than ever with emotional pitfalls.

Until puberty, girls and boys suffer from depression in about equal numbers. It isn't until sex hormones change the shape of our bodies and alter our internal chemistries that we suffer more than our male counterparts. As discussed in chapter 3, scientists are still unclear about how hormones and neurotransmitters interact to create this female vulnerability to mood disorders, but as millions of women can attest, they do, about once every month.

The Monthly Blues

The regulation of the menstrual cycle involves complex interactions among neurotransmitters and hormones. These interactions prompt a number of physical changes affecting almost every organ system in the body, including the brain. In particular, there appears to be a direct connection between hormones produced by the ovaries (estrogen and progesterone, the female sex hormones) and serotonin, the neurotransmitter most related to depression. In women who suffer from premenstrual syndrome, serotonin levels drop precipitously during the week before menstruation.

This serotonin depletion helps explain two common symptoms of PMS: mood swings and cravings for carbohydrates (substances that naturally boost serotonin levels in the brain). In fact, studies show that women with PMS eat an average of five hundred extra carbohydrate calories per day in the week or so before their periods.

Carolyn, a seventeen-year-old high school junior, describes her monthly bouts this way: "First comes the irritability and testiness about ten days before my period. That lasts about two or three days. Then I feel completely exhausted and sad, ready to cry at the drop of a hat, really. And I eat a lot, mostly pasta and sometimes chocolate, until my period starts."

Like many young women, Carolyn didn't realize that these feelings were part of a syndrome that can be treated. "Because I've been going through this monthly up-and-down thing since I was about eleven, I thought every girl felt this way. I didn't even mention it to my doctor until recently, when it started interfering with my schoolwork. We decided I'd try taking birth control pills to see if that evens out my moods. If it doesn't, I might try an antidepressant."

As you'll read later in this chapter, estrogen and progesterone may well help women who become depressed not only during their menstrual cycles, but also after giving birth or with menopause. The important thing to remember is that no woman, no matter her age, need suffer endlessly from unpleasant and undermining hormonal changes.

Marilyn, now a college sophomore, also began to struggle with her emotions during adolescence. "I don't how much my hormones have to do with my problems, but I do know things started going wrong when I was about fourteen, when I was a high school freshman. I remember starting that year with so much optimism: It was going to be perfect—I was going to be perfect. I'd be a cheerleader and make all honors and have a boyfriend. And I did, but what a price I paid. I'm still paying."

The Perfect Little Girl

One common response to the turmoil of adolescence, especially among teenaged girls, is perfectionism: to be the perfect little girl who pleases her parents, never makes a mistake, is the most beautiful, the smartest, the least trouble. This is especially true for girls who come from families troubled by alcoholism, physical abuse, or other turmoil.

"My father had an affair with another woman when I was twelve and my mom found out about it," Marilyn remembers. "They fought for three years—horrible, raging fights I can't believe they thought I didn't hear. Even though it was terrible, I didn't want my dad to leave. I know it sounds trite, but I really thought if I could be the perfect kid, he'd stick around. So I did whatever it took."

In Marilyn, the anxiety of her home life, combined with

her desire for perfection, developed into both chronic depression and an eating disorder she's struggled with ever since. "I started binging and purging when I was about fifteen. I was a cheerleader and popular and pretty, but I felt scared all the time, like at any moment somebody would discover that I was a fake, that my family was a mess. So I kept making all A's and going to all the parties and winning all my tennis matches. But I also had a secret life."

It wouldn't happen all the time, but once or twice a month, Marilyn would sneak loads of cookies, cakes, and pizza into her room, then eat everything in sight. "Then I'd go into the bathroom and throw up. I've been doing it, off and on, for years and no one has ever guessed. I only recently admitted it to my doctor."

As you can see, the drive for perfection can be a very dangerous thing. Experts see perfectionism as one of the biggest risk factors for depression and suicide, as well as for eating disorders. In fact, depression, eating disorders, and suicide appear to go hand in hand in many young adults. More than half of all bulimics have had a depressive episode disorder before the onset of the eating disorder, for instance, and more than 80 percent will experience an episode at some point in their lives. Twenty percent of bulimics and an even higher percentage of anorexics eventually make a suicide attempt.

Both perfectionism and eating disorders stem from a desperate desire to take control in a world that seems to be completely uncontrollable, especially for the average adolescent. Indeed, 86 percent of all eating disorders begin before the age of twenty. "I couldn't control what my parents did about their marriage, or what my friends thought about me," Marilyn remembers. "But I could control everything that happened to me: I *would* get all A's, I *would* make the all-star team, I *would* be the most popular girl in school. That I could control . . . until the emptiness would sneak up and then I'd have to eat and throw up. Afterward, I'd feel like a horrible failure for a few days, then make a pact with myself to take control again. A vicious cycle if there ever was one."

Eating disorders are not the only reactions to depression among young women. Some teenagers attempt to alleviate their feelings of low self-esteem and alienation by acting out. Some skip school or shoplift, others become sexually promiscuous. Still others may turn to drugs or alcohol abuse, both as a way of fitting in, and thus feeling less isolated, or to self-medicate.

Today, Marilyn takes medication and sees a therapist once a week. "I'm getting better. I'm beginning to set some realistic goals and to learn to forgive myself even if I don't meet them. I'm starting my junior year in the fall, and I want to be ready to make some decision about my career and how to shape it."

The Search for a Place in the World

Many young people on their own in their twenties are finding the real world a rather discouraging place to be—economically and emotionally. In 1996, the average twenty-five-year-old made about 20 percent less in real dollars than her counterpart made in 1976. According to the U.S. Census Bureau, the number of people under twenty-five who own their own home fell 46 percent and the number renting by themselves fell about 21 percent. More and more young adults leave college and head for home when they can't find a job in an increasingly shrinking and "downsizing" market. This often creates an undermining combination of stress, anxiety, and hopelessness.

Phoebe, who just celebrated her twenty-sixth birthday, received her Ph.D. in English literature, then immediately fell into a fullblown episode of anxiety and depression. "I moved into an apartment with my boyfriend and started looking for a job. I thought I'd teach or maybe go into advertising. I wasn't sure, but I thought everything would be okay. Then out of the blue, I began to have panic attacks. They were so bad I could barely leave my house. I missed a couple of interviews, then started going back to bed as soon as my boyfriend left for work. I'd get up just before he got home and pretend I'd had a full day. This went on for weeks."

Phoebe finally went to her family doctor, explaining only that she felt a little anxious. He put her on a mild tranquilizer and sent her home. "I don't know what happened, but a couple of weeks later I completely broke down. My boyfriend came home and found me curled up in my bed, sobbing uncontrollably. He called my parents, and we all went to the hospital. I stayed for two weeks until my depression and anxiety were brought under control. Now I can start to face whatever it is that's scaring me so—maybe it has to do with my boyfriend or settling down or finding a job. Maybe it's about all those things together."

As women pass from their late twenties into their thirties, the need to make decisions about their careers and family lives begins to gather even more momentum.

The Tentative Thirties

For most women today, life begins to take a much more definite shape during their thirties. Although we have more biological and social freedom than ever before, the need to make firm decisions about careers, marriage, and children tends to become more urgent as each year passes. For women who are psychologically or genetically vulnerable, depression and/or anxiety may creep in if expectations about these decisions are not met.

Jordan is a thirty-five-year-old writer who sought counseling after feeling "stuck and lazy," as she described it, for more than a year. "It started not when I turned thirty-five, like it's supposed to, but when I was about to turn thirty-four. I had all these expectations about where I'd be by the time I was thirty-five, and I suddenly realized I only had a year to go and there was no way I'd get there. No chance at all. I kind of just shut down."

Jordan talked her situation through with her therapist and discovered the source of her deep disappointment. "It wasn't that I thought I'd be married with children and a best-selling author by thirty-five. I just thought I'd be a whole lot closer to . . . something. Either success *or* a husband *or* . . . I don't know, a new goal maybe. I just didn't think there wouldn't be a man in sight, that I'd still be in debt, that I'd still be writing the same kind of stuff I wrote eight years ago, that everything would seem so static."

Depression and the Legacy of Abuse

Depression and anxiety came to Peri, a forty-three-year-old divorced woman, for a completely different set of reasons. Happy in her job as a legal secretary, asked by a man she loved to get married, Peri thought she was about to make her dreams come true until the nightmares came.

"I started having these horrible dreams, vague at first. I'd wake up and not remember anything, but feel dreadful shame and fear. They started recurring, every week or so, then more often. It got to be I was too scared to sleep," Peri recalls. "Then memories of my grandfather and me sitting on the porch swing would flash in front of me at the oddest times. I couldn't figure it out—I hadn't thought of him in years—but I felt the same terror I did when I woke up from the nightmares."

Posttraumatic stress disorder, or PTSD, was first designated as a psychiatric disorder in 1980 after large numbers of American Vietnam War veterans developed troubling symptoms after returning home. What scientists know now is that any traumatic event that threatened one's life or safety can cause PTSD, including physical or sexual abuse.

"I didn't know what to do. I couldn't get close to my boyfriend, and I didn't know why," Peri admits. "I couldn't stand to be touched. At first I thought it was because I loved him too much and was afraid I'd ruin my second marriage the way I'd ruined the first. Or that I didn't deserve his love for some reason. I couldn't sleep, I couldn't eat. Finally, I went to my doctor and got some help."

After alleviating the worst of the depressive and anxious symptoms with medication, Peri slowly but surely retrieved long-buried memories of being fondled by her grandfather. She realized that the abuse had been slowly eating away at her since it happened, more than thirty years before.

"I've read a lot about depression and anxiety, and I know a lot has to do with brain chemistry," Peri says. "I know this isn't scientifically correct, but I think that somehow horrible memories might act like a poison, killing brain cells or neurotransmitters or whatever. And that's why you can become so depressed without knowing the reason why."

No one knows exactly what causes PTSD or the depression that so often travels with it, but Peri's idea may have more merit than she imagines. While it's not the memories themselves that are the poison, it could well be the stress it takes to bury those memories that causes the chemical disruption leading to depression. We do know that high rates of depression exist in both adolescents and adult women who've been sexually abused as children.

More than the Baby Blues

Like Peri, Gail began to feel sad and anxious just when she thought she had everything in the world she'd always wanted. In her case, depression draped over her world two months after her son was born. We've all heard about "the baby blues," the sadness and anxiety that sneaks up on about half of all new mothers. Scientists think this fairly common dip in mood is probably related to the dramatic hormonal changes—mainly the withdrawal of progesterone and estrogen—that occur following childbirth. Within a few weeks or so, most women return to normal without the need for intervention.

In about 10 percent of new mothers, however, full-blown postpartum depression sets in. The symptoms frequently start about two to three weeks after the woman gives birth and peak at about three months. Unless she gets help, postpartum depression can easily linger, worsen, or, as it did in Gail's case, become complicated by anxiety or another emotional illness.

What's the difference between women with "normal" baby blues and those who develop postpartum depression? No one really knows. It could be that women with postpartum depression are overly sensitive to hormonal fluctuations, as is true for women who experience PMS. It also appears that hormones other than estrogen and progesterone, including thyroid hormone and cortisol, also may become unbalanced in these women. Still another theory is that the body's internal clock is knocked off its regular schedule by these hormonal changes—as well as by the unpredictable sleep patterns that a new mother must endure—leaving the body, mind, and soul feeling out-of-sync and disconcerted.

Because Gail weaned her son a few months ago, she's able to take medication—both an antianxiety drug called

Klonopin and an antidepressant. She's also seeing a therapist to help her sort through some of the emotional issues that might have contributed to her depression. "I knew it would be hard, of course, to be a mother," Gail admits. "But I didn't realize how much I'd love my son, how scared I was that something could happen to him. At the same time, I know I miss my job, my friends, having a social life. And I feel guilty about that, too. But I'm lucky. I have a supportive husband who helps as much as he can. I know not everyone does."

Motherhood Without Marriage: A Recipe for Stress

"Overwhelmed and very, very sad and scared. That's the way I feel now," thirty-eight-year-old Rebecca admits. "I have a fourteen-month-old baby, a full-time job, and my heart's been broken. I'm not sure how much more I can take."

Rebecca is one of the increasing number of women who decide to become single mothers. "I never thought it would come to this. It's not like I heard the clock ticking and just ran out and got pregnant. I was in a loving relationship with a man who didn't want to get married, wasn't even sure he ever wanted a family. When I got pregnant—an accident—I thought I could bring him around, that eventually he'd see the joy in all this. And, the truth is, I was almost thirty-seven years old and I wasn't sure I'd get another chance to get pregnant. The guy left. I kept the baby. I didn't think it'd be easy to raise a child alone, but I had no idea how hard it would really be."

Single motherhood is on the rise, and has been since the 1980s. The National Center for Health Statistics reports that from 1980 to 1988 the birth rate jumped 69 percent for unmarried white women—and the largest increases occurred among women over twenty-five years of age. No one knows exactly how much more at risk for depression single mothers are than their married counterparts. However, it seems likely that the increased stress levels under which they live might serve to upset their mental and physical well-being, especially if they are genetically or psychologically predisposed.

It is difficult to measure how much stress *not* being able to have a child, either due to infertility or circumstances, puts on the average woman who longs to be a mother. But we do know that the biological clock does, in fact, tick louder and longer than ever before, well into a woman's forties and even her fifties. And it isn't counting down the time left just to have a child, but also to find a clear and happy path through the rest of one's life.

Consolidating in the Forties

"The thing about turning forty is that while you might not feel middle-aged, you are. Chances are, half your life is over. It came as a big shock to me. Shook me to my core, really." Julia, who's been in therapy since an episode of depression overwhelmed her a year ago, remembers the onset of the disease. "I looked at my life, and all I could hear were the lines in that song by the Talking Heads: 'Is this my beautiful life? Is this my beautiful house?' when I talked to my mother about it, she smiled this sad smile, and remembered thinking almost the same thing when she turned thirty-five, but for her, the song was 'Is That All There Is?'"

The realization that where you are now is not where you want to be can come at any time. After all, it hit Jordan at thirty-four. But when it occurs in your forties, it can have a greater sense of finality. Julia put it this way, "I felt awful. I thought, not only do I not have what I thought I'd have, but what I do have, I'm stuck with for the rest of my life."

Women who delay childbirth until their early forties, as many more every day choose to do, may find the burdens of motherhood—or the pain of newly discovered infertility—to be especially challenging. Claudia, who suffered a miscarriage two years ago at the age of thirty-nine, worries that she's had difficulty conceiving since then because she feels ambivalent about becoming a mother at forty-two or older.

"My husband and I tried for three years before I got pregnant last time. We were devastated by the miscarriage, and we've been trying to get pregnant ever since," Claudia explains. "But somehow my heart really isn't in it. I feel lost, guilty, stuck, panicked all at once. I wonder if somehow that's keeping me from getting pregnant."

In addition to seeing a therapist on her own, Claudia attends counseling with her husband. Together, they're trying to plan a different kind of future together than either one of them had imagined. "I guess it's hard to readjust my expectations at this point. Since I was a kid, I pictured my future in a certain way, and a child was at the center of it. Now, I don't know what to expect, and that's what's got me so shook up."

Having unmet expectations—and the fear that you have nothing that can replace or supplant them—is one of the most troubling and stressful challenges for the increasing numbers of women turning forty and fifty today. For some, this stress can trigger an addiction to alcohol or drugs or cause an existing dependence to deepen.

Face to Face with Addiction

"I hid my drinking problem from everyone, even myself," Julia confesses. "Maybe it wasn't a problem earlier, before this depression really set in. But then again, I don't know. Alcohol has always been a part of my life—an important part."

Women, alcohol, and depression often form a tragic triangle. Both alcoholism and depression have genetic components, and they often run together through families. Approximately 40 percent of all adults who abuse alcohol and drugs are women; more than 70 percent of women at the Betty Ford Center visit the treatment center for alcohol addiction. According to studies conducted by the National Institute of Mental Health, half of women alcoholics are seriously depressed and two-thirds of them are depressed before they begin abusing alcohol.

"I don't know which came first, to tell the truth," Julia says. "Maybe I've been ... what do they call it? ... 'self-medicating' for years. I know I've had my ups and downs, and periods when I know I drank too much. Now I know it's become a problem. I hide how much I drink from my husband, I drink when I'm alone, and I can't seem to stop."

With help and encouragement from a therapist, Julia is facing her addiction to alcohol for the first time. She realizes that her feelings of disappointment about her life may well be clouded by alcohol, and by the disease of depression itself.

"I know I have to take care of this now, before it's too late," Julia relates. "I want the second half of my life to be as good—maybe even better—than the first."

Forging the Passage

Just a few decades ago, fifty marked the beginning of the end of your life. Today, as Gail Sheehy puts it in her book *New Passages*, many men and women enter a second adulthood, one filled with exciting new goals and opportunities. You may reach a new level of power and confidence in your career at this time, or perhaps embark on a new one.

If you're financially secure, you might be thinking of taking early retirement and exploring other aspects of life.

As exciting as this time may be, however, it can also be fraught with uncertainty and change. Although menopause—which occurs at the average age of fifty-one—doesn't cause depression in most women, it does set up certain vulnerabilities, both biological and psychological. The signs of aging are more certain now. The truth is, for most of us the transition between young and old can occur in the blink of an eye. It can happen when your last parent dies and you realize you're the head of your family. Or maybe your child having a child marks the turning point. Whenever it happens, it may set off a chain reaction of fear, anxiety, and depression.

The Empty Nest

Beth, a woman in her early fifties who's suffered with bouts of depression throughout her life, experienced her worst one yet when her youngest daughter left for college. "My husband and I divorced eight years ago, but I still had my daughter. I also cared for my mother, who had Parkinson's disease until she died last year. Then when Sandy left for school, I froze. I was alone. I was old. I was scared."

In therapy and on medication, Beth is learning to reach out in new directions in order to fill her life in a positive way. She now volunteers at a local soup kitchen and contemplates doing some freelance marketing work. She's excited about creating a "second adulthood" that will keep her as young, vital, and content as possible—for as long as possible, even as she ages.

Heading into Late Life

"My mother has been troubled by bouts of depression for as long as I can remember," admits thirty-four-year-old Robert about his sixty-six-year-old mother, Marjorie. "But the last year or so, it's been terrible. Everything caught up with her all at once, it seems. My father died two years ago, because of her age she's being pushed aside at work, and her doctor recently diagnosed her with diabetes. She's feeling old, alone. . . . It's really disturbing her."

Contrary to the way she feels now, Marjorie is far from alone in her situation. According to the National Institutes of Health, about 6 million of the 32 million Americans sixty-five and older suffer from some level of clinical depression. At least 50 to 75 percent go undiagnosed.

The risks for suicide with untreated depression in the elderly are enormous. Some physicians fear that severe depression can lead some elderly patients to make deadly, inappropriate decisions about continuation of medical treatment. If someone is depressed, it is much more likely that she will choose to reject medical care she might otherwise have accepted if her depression were treated.

One study, conducted at the Portland Veterans Administration Medical Center and reported in the November 1994 *American Journal of Psychiatry*, supports the idea that in many depressed persons, hopelessness, pessimism, and excessive emphasis on the burdens of treatment temporarily alter someone's ability to objectively weigh the risks and benefits of medical treatment. Furthermore, it's logical to assume that if you're depressed, you'll be much less likely to take medication, perform physical therapy, or otherwise participate in a healthy lifestyle. For some, these lapses in self-care may be a covert suicidal act—one that requires and deserves medical attention.

The Challenge of Diagnosis

Only recently has depression among the elderly been widely recognized as a serious and common health problem, and there remains a great deal of ignorance about it among health care professionals as well as the general public. Indeed, studies of elderly people who committed suicide as a result of depression show that about 75 percent visited a doctor within a week of their deaths, but in only 25 percent of those cases did the doctor recognize that the patient was depressed.

Part of the difficulty stems from a misunderstanding of the aging process. Marjorie's son, Robert, only recognized his mother's problem as psychiatric in nature because she had been depressed in the past. Most of us have been brought up to think of mood disturbances as being a natural part of the aging process. It's normal, we think, for older people to become discouraged and sad. After all, they're nearing the end of their lives.

The truth, however, is that the personality does not change in any fundamental way as we age. If someone has always been relatively happy and well-adjusted, symptoms of depression are not normal and should be assessed by a health professional—a course of action many older people are loath to take.

Indeed, perhaps more than younger people, women turning seventy today still believe that depression is a character flaw and not an illness. They are so convinced that their problems are not emotional in nature that they develop physical symptoms, like headaches, stomachaches, and other very real illnesses that are actually psychological in origin.

"I didn't really think I was depressed," Gloria says. "I thought I was getting sick. It was because my doctor was sensitive to the signs of depression in someone my age that he referred me to a psychiatrist."

In someone healthy and lucid like Gloria, a diagnosis of depression is relatively easy to make. It becomes much more difficult, however, when Alzheimer's disease or another form of dementia is also present. Between 17 and 50 percent of elderly patients may experience a combination of dementia and depression, and both conditions require treatment. Other medical conditions common to the aging population, including heart disease and Parkinson's disease, may also cause depressive symptoms. The good news is that depression in later life can be treated successfully, even if there are medical complications.

TREATMENT OPTIONS ABOUND

Millions of people every year live in the quiet desperation of dysthymia or the deep darkness of a major depression. The vast majority of them do so needlessly. Although depression is a serious disorder, it is also one of the most treatable. No matter your age or your stage of life, if you're depressed, there's help for you out there.

As discussed in chapter 1, it isn't always easy to seek help for a problem like depression. "I never in my life thought I'd see a psychiatrist," eighty-two-year-old Gloria admits. "In my day, it wasn't something you did—unless you were very rich or very crazy!" But when faced with having to move out of the family home she'd inhabited for more than fifty years and with an increasingly intransigent yet passive husband, Gloria sought help for the depression that ensued.

"What my doctor taught me was how to think about my situation differently. Instead of resenting all the work I had to do to keep my husband and myself on the right track, I saw my resourcefulness and determination as positive qualities. I saw the move to a smaller place as an opportunity—to travel, to spend our savings more freely, to have some fun. As for my husband, well, I've had to deal with the way he is for sixty years, I might as well keep going!"

Gloria broke through her depression with the help of her therapist. Together they decided that Gloria did not need to take an antidepressant or other psychotherapeutic drug. Many others with depression, however, require a combination of medication and psychotherapy in order to manage their disease and alleviate symptoms.

"I wouldn't have had it in me to even drive to my therapy sessions had I not been on medication," admits Cynthia, a sixty-four-year-old woman who began to suffer from severe depression following her daughter's unexpected death in a boating accident. "I was so griefstricken when my daughter died, and then work began to go badly. Because of my age, I felt pressure to quit a job I really needed. A wave of darkness just flooded me. It felt like something simply sapped all my strength, all my will away. I couldn't sleep, couldn't manage my finances, nothing got done at all. I very nearly lost my job. My doctor gave me an antidepressant and a few weeks later I had energy for the first time in years. It didn't solve all of my problems, not by a long shot. But it gave me the ability to try again."

Deciding on a Course of Treatment

Like Gloria, Cynthia, and the other women you've met so far in this book, you too can find the help you need to feel better. Indeed, you've taken the first giant step toward recovery simply by picking up this book and reading this far.

Once a mental health professional diagnoses your depression (see chapter 2 for more information), you and your therapist then can decide upon the most appropriate course of treatment. The severity of your disease, your current health and health history, and your personal needs and priorities are the main factors considered during this process. Generally speaking, treatment for depression has four main goals:

1. To restore any underlying chemical imbalance in the brain
2. To help you sort through any personal issues, past or present, that may contribute to or complicate your condition
3. To help you repair any relationship or situation that may have been damaged during your bout with depression
4. To teach you new, more positive ways to think about yourself and to better manage your life and relationships

In chapter 6, you'll read about the various types of psychotherapy available to help you break through the blanket of despair and take control of your life in a more positive and active way. And, as you may know from personal experience, depression affects not only the individual with the disease but family, work, and social relationships as well. That's a subject discussed in both chapters 6 and 7.

Next, chapter 5 explores the medication now available to treat depression, as well as the circumstances under which hospitalization and/or electroconvulsive therapy might be helpful. In addition to descriptions of the effects and side effects of many common antidepressants, you'll also find information about taking medication safely and how to assess its effectiveness.

IMPORTANT QUESTIONS AND ANSWERS ABOUT CHAPTER 4

Q. I'm forty-eight years old and worried about menopause. Does menopause mean automatic depression?

A. Not at all. Many women pass through menopause with few or no mood changes. In fact, a study done by the Eastern Baltimore Mental Health Unit during the early 1980s showed that people between the ages of eighteen and sixty-four had three times the incidence of depression than those in the sixty-five to seventy-four age group.

However, it is true that the drop in estrogen and progesterone does cause mood swings and irritability in some women—at least for a short time. Treatment with estrogen and progesterone (hormone replacement therapy or HRT) may help alleviate these symptoms. In addition, HRT may also alleviate other unpleasant symptoms of menopause that can trigger depression. Hot flashes, for instance, can become so severe that a woman feels trapped by them. Or they can occur at night so often that sleep patterns are disrupted, leading to depressive symptoms. If you feel you might benefit from taking HRT, talk to your doctor. He or she can help you put your mind at ease about the upcoming changes in your body.

Q. When does grief become depression? My father died about a year ago, and my mother still barely leaves the house and often cries at the drop of a hat. They were married for fifty-five years, and I don't think she wants to go on.

A. There is no easy dividing line between grief and depression. Grief takes time and energy to pass through, and the amount of time and energy differs with each individual. It may be natural for your mother to need more time to mourn the loss of her life-long companion, and she needs your continued support during this painful time. However, if you are concerned that your mother is neglecting her health in any way, or has become stuck in the grieving process for too long, you should gently suggest that she visit a therapist or a support group of some kind.

5
▼

THE MEDICAL TREATMENT OF DEPRESSION

"I resisted taking medication for a long, long time, even after my suicide attempt," admits Beth, a fifty-one-year-old woman who has suffered with depression and dysthymia for most of her life. "I remember saying to my therapist, 'But Glenn, how will I know if I'm feeling better because of the medication or because my life is really getting better?' I'll never forget what he said to me: 'Beth, what does it matter? You'll *feel* better, which is what's most important now. Then you can take a look at your life with more objectivity.' I took his advice and three weeks later, I had a little energy and inspiration, and could start to figure out how to fix what needed fixing."

Beth speaks for virtually millions of women who have found relief with the help of antidepressants. Medication appears to greatly improve symptoms of depression in about 80 percent of the people who take them. For those living the chronic "underlife" of dysthymia, antidepressants can reignite a long dormant spark for living. For those with major depression, medication can literally save lives.

"I really came close to suicide," admits Marjorie, the sixty-six-year-old woman with psychotic depression you met in chapter 4. "If my son hadn't gotten me to a doctor, I'm not sure I would have survived."

As we'll discuss later, Marjorie was treated first with ECT (electroconvulsive therapy) to more quickly alleviate her severe depression. Her doctor then placed her on an antidepressant. "I was a little nervous about taking medication, but I'd never want to feel like I did before. I do think the medicine is helping me to stay vital and strong."

That said, it's important to point out that while antidepressant medication is effective for the vast majority of women with depression, it is not a panacea or a miracle cure. First, there is a small minority of people—about 10 percent—for whom medication appears to have little effect. Second, anyone who develops depression is likely to have some issues in her personal life that need addressing with psychotherapy. Just as aspirin reduces a fever without clearing up the infection that causes it, psychotropic medications act by controlling symptoms but do not "cure" depression. Instead, they lessen their burden and help make psychotherapy more effective.

"There's no question that taking Prozac keeps me stable and energized," Marilyn says. "But I have a lot of problems that I know contribute to my depression and my bulimia. There's stuff I need to work out about my childhood—I know, who doesn't?—and I know I have negative thought patterns that really screw me up. My therapist helps me with that, while the Prozac keeps me going."

In chapter 6, we discuss the benefits of therapy in greater depth. In the meantime, let's explore what is often the first line of treatment for many cases of major depression and dysthymia—medication.

ANTIDEPRESSANT MEDICATION: THE WHYS AND WHEREFORES

Even today, as we head toward the twenty-first century, there remains a great deal of skepticism over, and disdain for, psychotherapeutic drugs of any kind. For many of the same reasons that men and women resist seeing a therapist, they also resist taking medication. Some feel special shame that their emotional problems require drug therapy. Others, like Beth, believe that even if medication makes you feel better, it doesn't really count. Others worry, usually needlessly, about unwanted side effects.

Fortunately, we've now had more than three decades of experience with antidepressant drugs and we know that, for the most part, they are quite safe. Their side effects are usually mild and tend to subside after a few weeks or months. We also know that they work for the vast majority of men and women suffering from depression, alleviating their symptoms and considerably shortening the course of the disease.

What we don't know is exactly how and why these medications work. As discussed in Chapter 3, the intricate workings of the brain and endocrine system remain somewhat of a mystery. Brain chemistry—the production and function of neurotransmitters—is particularly complex, and it is only in the last few decades that scientists have learned enough about it to design drugs that help to restore any imbalances that occur.

Three types of drugs—each of which works to fine-tune the balance of neurotransmitters in a slighly different way—have been found to be most effective in treating depression: *selective serotonin reuptake inhibitors* (SSRIs), *tricyclic antidepressants* (TCAs), and *monoamine oxidase inhibitors* (MAOIs). There are also some drugs like bupropion (Wellbutrin), nefazodone (Serzone), and trazodone

(Desyrel), that are unrelated to the others but are known to help alleviate depression. When depression is complicated by other psychological disorders, such as posttraumatic stress or anxiety, other drugs may be used alone or in combination with an antidepressant. *Benzodiazepines* are the most commonly used antianxiety drugs.

Later in this chapter, we describe the specific uses, benefits, and side effects of these drugs in further depth. In the end, however, all medication used to treat depression and related disorders has the same goal: to provide the brain with the raw materials it needs to send and receive proper messages about mood and behavior.

Before You Decide to Take Medication

Although antidepressants are usually quite safe, they are nonetheless strong drugs that alter the workings of your brain and body. It is important that you consider the matter thoroughly with both your therapist and the doctor who prescribes the medication, if your therapist is not a medical doctor. Here are some issues to discuss with your doctor as you're deciding about drug therapy.

▼ *Make sure you tell your doctor about any other medication you take.*

Phoebe, a twenty-six-year-old woman with anxiety and depresssion, was surprised to find that the birth control pills she took might interefere with an antianxiety medication. Because Beth took antihistamines to alleviate her allergies, her doctor decided against prescribing one antidepressant because of its potential to cause a harmful drug interaction.

Any medication—even an over-the-counter drug—has the potential to modify your body chemistry and thus exacerbate an underlying health problem. In addition, there are certain drugs that may be dangerous when taken in combination with one another or when taken with alcohol, or, in some cases, with certain kinds of food. Before prescribing medication, your doctor should study your medical history and check your current health status to make sure you don't have a medical condition that would be adversely affected by antidepressant medication. It's up to you to tell him or her about every drug—prescription or over-the-counter—that you take. This information will allow your doctor to prescribe the safest and most effective medication for you.

▼ *Tell your doctor if you feel you have a problem with alcohol or other substances.*

It is absolutely essential that you tell your doctor if you are addicted to alcohol or any so-called recreational drug. Statistics show that between 10 and 30 percent of alcoholics become depressed over time and the number is even higher for those with drug dependencies. As discussed in chapter 4, some researchers believe that many people develop an addiction to alcohol or drugs as a way to "self-medicate"—to deaden the pain of their depression by, biochemically speaking, attempting to correct a chemical imbalance in the brain.

If you feel you have a problem, you must get help for both your substance abuse problem and your depression. It is impossible to successfully treat one without dealing with the other. In one study, 60 percent of people admitted to a particular alcohol treatment program suffered with coexisting depression, but only 10 percent were prescribed an antidepressant. A year later, those whose depression was left untreated were both still drinking and still depressed.

Depending on the severity of your addiction, your general health, and other considerations, your doctor may decide that you should enter a substance abuse treatment center or detoxify on an outpatient basis before starting treatment for depression. Most antidepressants have the potential to cause serious, sometimes fatal, side effects if taken with alcohol or other drugs.

If your substance abuse problem is relatively mild, and you feel you can stop drinking on your own or in combination with a program like Alcoholics Anonymous, then your doctor may decide to treat your depression with medication as well as psychotherapy relatively soon. As is true for so much about depression, a decision like this one is highly dependent on individual circumstances and can only be made after your doctor performs a careful psychological and physical examination.

▼ *Find out all you can about every medication you take.*

Since depression often coexists with other psychiatric disorders, your doctor may decide to treat you with more than one drug. For each drug your doctor prescribes, ask and receive answers to the following questions. We answer some of these questions in a general way later in the chapter.

—What is the name of the medication and how does it work?

—How and when do I take it, and when do I stop taking it?

—What foods, drinks, other medications, or activities should I avoid while taking this medication?

—What are the side effects and what should I do if they occur?

—What should I do if I forget to take my medicine?

—How will I know if the medicine is working?

—How long will I have to take the medicine?

—Is there any risk that I could become addicted?

—Can you provide me with any written information about the medication?

—How much does the medication cost?

Listen carefully to your doctor's answers, and take notes on important points. Read all written material provided by your doctor or that comes with the prescription itself. Follow all directions with care. Always remember that you have a right to know everything about the drugs you take and their expected effects and side effects. Armed with this information, you'll be able to make an informed decision, based on a full understanding of the risks and benefits, about whether or not drug treatment is right for you.

▼ *Remember at all times that you are in control of your therapy.*

Many people fear that by deciding to take antidepressants they are somehow giving control of their minds over to the drugs or to the doctor. Nothing could be further from the truth. By reestablishing the proper connections among the neurons in your brain, an antidepressant in effect hands the controls back to you.

Unless you are terribly ill and incapacitated, you remain in charge of your own recovery from depression— whether or not you decide to take medication. If there ever comes a time when you feel that medication is not right for you, just let your therapist know. Unless your health would be seriously impaired, it is highly likely that he or she would accede to your wishes and taper off your medication appropriately.

Choosing an Antidepressant

Which drug or combination of drugs works for any given individual depends largely upon her own particular brain chemistry and constellation of symptoms. Some people may respond better to one medication than another. Since no test exists to measure exactly how one's brain chemistry is imbalanced or why it became that way, prescribing an antidepressant is often a hit-or-miss affair. Your doctor will decide which drug is best for you based on an evaluation of your symptoms, medical history, and current co-existing physical or psychological problems.

However, it's important that you be as patient and flexible as possible. In taking an antidepressant, you are attempting to reestablish a proper balance of neurotransmitters in your brain. Needless to say, that's a pretty tricky enterprise that often requires a bit of finesse from your doctor and a great deal of patience on your part. It may take a few tries before you find the drug or combination of drugs that works for you.

In addition to these general guidelines, there are some further special considerations:

▼ *If you are trying to conceive, are pregnant, or are nursing:* The question of initiating or continuing antidepressants when you are planning to become pregnant, carrying a child, or breast-feeding remains a difficult one. Most physicians urge that women take no medication at all during pregnancy, unless their depression is life-threatening. Discuss the matter thoroughly with your physician if you have any concerns.

▼ *If you are over 70:* In most cases, doctors will prescribe lower dosages of certain antidepressants (specifically the tricyclics) for older patients, especially those with known cardiac conditions. Electroconvulsive therapy (ECT) is often used on severely depressed elders who are unable to tolerate antidepressants of any kind.

After evaluating your symptoms and individual health profile, your doctor will decide which among the many medication options to try first. Depending on a variety of factors, your doctor may decide to test your blood and perform metabolic studies on a regular basis to determine the effect the drug has on you. Following is a brief guide to the most commonly used medications for treating depression and related disorders.

A Guide to Drugs Used to Treat Depression

ANTIDEPRESSANTS

As discussed, antidepressants work to restore a proper balance of neurotransmitters in the brain, thereby allowing messages about mood and behavior to be delivered and received. They do so by acting to increase the available amount of the serotonin, norepinephrine, and, to a lesser degree, dopamine.

There are three classes of antidepressants: selective serotonin reuptake inhibitors, tricyclic antidepressants, and monoamine oxidase inhibitors. Let's take them one by one.

Selective Serotonin Reuptake Inhibitors

SSRIs are the newest of the three main categories of antidepressants. As their name implies, they work to relieve depression by selectively inhibiting the reuptake (reabsorption) of the neurotransmitter serotonin. The older antidepressants, called tricyclics, block the reuptake of both serotonin and norepinephrine. When too much norepinephrine exists in the brain, side effects like dry mouth and dizziness occur that SSRIs generally avoid. Prozac is the most well-known and commonly prescribed SSRI.

SSRIs are often prescribed for the elderly because of their lack of side effects like orthostatic hypotension, a sudden drop in blood pressure that causes dizziness and—potentially—a dangerous fall. They are also often the best choice for women with medical problems such as heart disease, dementia, or Alzheimer's disease, and certain other mental disorders such as bulimia or posttraumatic stress disorder.

General side effects: SSRIs may cause side effects in some individuals. They can cause nervousness or, conversely, drowsiness, sleep problems, headaches, weight gain or loss, as well as nausea and other gastrointestinal symptoms. Perhaps one of the most troubling side effects, and one that affects about 10 to 20 percent of women who use SSRIs, is sexual dysfunction, including decreased sexual desire and delayed orgasm. Finally, SSRIs must never be used in combination with MAOIs (monoamine oxidase inhibitors). Such a combination can cause serious, sometimes fatal reactions.

FLUOXETINE (PROZAC)

Dosage: 10 to 20 mg per day once a day to start. If there is no improvement in two to three weeks, the dose can be increased by 10 to 20 mg/day up to a maximum of 60 mg per day.

Special Considerations: Fluoxetine tends to be the most stimulating of the SSRIs and therefore may not be advised for someone recovering from a heart attack. Because it may interefere with the liver's ability to metabolize certain other drugs, taking fluoxetine may heighten the effects of other medication. Fluoxetine stays in the body for a long time—just one dose can take up to fourteen days to disappear.

FLUVOXAMINE (LUVOX)

Dosage: 50 mg once a day up to 200 mg in two daily dosages of 100 mg each.

Special Considerations: Fluvoxamine is also used to treat obsessive-compulsive disorder and is therefore most helpful in patients who also suffer from anxiety disorders. It also may be more sedating than other SSRIs, so your doctor may suggest you take fluvoxamine at nighttime.

PAROXETINE (PAXIL)

Dosage: 10 to 20 mg per day once a day up to a maximum of 50 mg per day.

Special Considerations: Paroxetine may cause headaches, nausea, dry mouth, and drowsiness. Paroxetine tends to be slightly less stimulating than fluoxetine and does not stay in the body nearly as long, only about one day.

SERTRALINE (ZOLOFT)

Dosage: 25 to 50 mg per day up to a 100 mg per day.

Special Considerations: Sertraline usually produces less nervousness than fluoxetine and may interfere less with the action of other drugs.

VENLAFAZINE (EFFEXOR)

Dosage: 75 to 225 mg per day, given in two or three divided doses. Dosages as high as 375 mg per day have been used in patients with serious depression.

Special Considerations: In rare cases, venlafaxine causes a rise in blood pressure, which may make this medication less desirable for women with hypertension or other cardiac problems.

Tricyclic Antidepressants

Prescribed since the 1950s, tricyclic antidepressants (also called TCAs) were among the first drugs developed to treat depression. By slowing the rate of reuptake, they raise the levels of the neurotransmitters serotonin and norepinephrine.

General side effects: Weight gain is a common side effect of tricyclics; some women put on several pounds while using the drug. Tricyclics also may cause dizziness or confusion, especially at the beginning of treatment. Flushing, sweating, allergic skin reactions, speech impairment, and anxiety are less common side effects.

The most serious side effects of tricyclic antidepressants are cardiac-related. That's because they block the action of a neurotransmitter called acetylcholine, which causes such side effects as blurred vision, dry mouth, constipation, orthostatic hypotension (feeling dizzy when standing up due to a sudden, temporary drop in blood pressure), increased sweating, difficulty urinating, changes in sexual desire or ability, fatigue, and weakness. Because TCAs may create cardiovascular problems, women with a history of heart disease should avoid them. Tricyclics can interact with any medications that affect the central nervous system, including allergy drugs, muscle relaxants, and sleeping pills, which is why it's important to tell your doctor about any medication you take.

Please note that each tricyclic works a little differently, and thus may cause slightly different side effects as well. Amitriptyline (Elavil), for instance, may make you feel drowsy, while desipramine (Norpramin) often has the opposite effect, causing you to feel anxious and restless.

Caution: Tricyclic overdoses—intentional and unintentional— can and do occur. Symptoms of an overdose of tricyclics generally develop within an hour and may include rapid heartbeat, dilated pupils, flushed face, and agitation. Confusion, loss of consciousness, seizures, cardiorespiratory collapse, and death may occur if left untreated.

AMITRIPTYLINE (ELAVIL, ENDEP)

Dosage: 50 to 75 mg per day up to 150 mg or 250 mg per day.

Special Considerations: Amitriptyline tends to be the most sedating of all antidepressants and is thus especially useful at night as a sleep aid. It is not often prescribed for elderly patients, since it can cause memory problems and confusion.

DESIPRAMINE (NORPRAMIN, PERTOFRANE)

Dosage: 50 to 75 mg per day up to 150 mg per day or in some cases 200 to 300 mg per day.

Special Considerations: Desipramine tends to be less sedating and more stimulating than other tricyclics, and may cause anxiety, restlessness, and muscle twitches in some people. On the other hand, it also is less likely to cause weight gain.

DOXEPIN (ADAPIN, SINEQUAN)

Dosage: 50 to 75 mg per day up to 150 to 300 mg per day.

Special Considerations: Like amitriptyline, doxepin should be taken at night since it often has a powerful sedating effect.

IMIPRAMINE (TOFRANIL, JANIMINE)

Dosage: 50 to 75 mg per day up to 150 to 300 mg per day.

Special Considerations: Imipramine is known to produce most of the typical side effects of tricyclic antidepressants.

NORTRIPTYLINE (AVENTYL, PAMELOR)

Dosage: 25 to 50 mg per day up to a maximum of 150 mg per day.

Special Considerations: Nortriptyline is especially useful for patients with depression and panic or other anxiety disorders.

Monoamine Oxidase Inhibitors (MAOIs)

MAOIs work by inhibiting an enzyme called monoamine oxidase from breaking down neurotransmitters like serotonin and norepinephrine. Because they necessitate severe dietary restrictions, MAOIs are not usually first-line treatments for depression. They also can have very toxic—even fatal—interactions with other medications. However, if a patient has been unable to tolerate or has failed to respond to SSRIs and tricyclics, then MAOI treatment might be indicated. MAOIs may be helpful for some women with atypical depression, that is, sleeping and eating more than usual and feeling anxious.

General side effects: MAOIs cause similar side effects to those of other antidepressants. They also react with certain foods and alcoholic beverages (such as aged cheeses, foods containing monosodium glutamate (MSG), Chianti and other red wines) and other medications (including over-the-counter cold and allergy preparations, local anesthetics, amphetamines, antihistamines, insulin, narcotics, anti-Parkinson's disease medication, and some antidepressants (particularly the SSRIs). If you and your doctor decide an MAOI is best for you, make sure he or she provides you with a list of foods and medications to avoid—and follow it to the letter!

PHENELZINE (NARDIL)

Dosage: 15 to 30 mg per day up to 45 to 75 mg per day.
Special Considerations: Phenelzine has a cumulative effect, which means that the doctor may cut the dosage after a period of time. This drug is extremely dangerous when combined with cocaine and cocaine-related drugs, and can cause serious adverse affects when used with Novocain or general anesthesia.

TRANYLCYPROMINE (PARNATE)

Dosage: 20 mg per day taken in two 10 mg doses.
Special Considerations: Parnate may cause restlessness and agitation.

Atypical Antidepressants

Some medications used to treat depression are chemically different from the three main classes of antidepressants. New drugs are being developed every day, but for now the four most common atypical antidepressants are bupropion (Wellbutrin), which may target the neurotransmitter dopamine; trazadone (Desyrel), which targets serotonin receptors; nefazodone (Serzone), which blocks a specific serotonin receptor subtype; and venlafaxine (Effexor), which works by blocking the reuptake of both serotonin and norepinephrine, but with fewer side effects than tricyclics.

BUPROPION (WELLBUTRIN)

Dosage: 100 mg twice a day up to 300 mg or a maximum dose of 450 mg per day. No dose should exceed 150 mg and there should be intervals of at least four hours between doses.

Special Considerations: Wellbutrin is usually very well tolerated, causing fewer side effects than most other antidepressants. The risk for weight gain, drowsiness, and sexual dysfunction is much lower than for most other antidepressants. It does, however, cause seizures in a small minority of people—about 4 in every 1,000 who take it. Seizures are more likely to occur at high doses. Like SSRIs, bupropion cannot be used in combination with MAOIs.

TRAZADONE (DESYREL)

Dosage: 50 to 100 mg per day when used in combination with an SSRI; 50 to 100 mg per day taken in two doses.

Special Considerations: Trazadone is a highly sedating antidepressant, which makes it useful for people with sleep problems who take it at night. It also appears to alleviate sexual dysfunction in women who develop such problems with SSRIs. It may cause side effects such as dry mouth, constipation, and postural hypotension.

NEFAZODONE (SERZONE)

Dosage: 200 mg per day, given in two separate doses.

Special Considerations: Like other SSRIs, nefazodone tends not to cause anxiety or drowsiness. Nefazodone should not be taken by patients using MAOIs.

ANTIANXIETY MEDICATIONS

Someone who suffers from a combination of depression and anxiety may be prescribed an antidepressant first if the depressive symptoms are worse, and an antianxiety medication if the anxiety symptoms are more troubling. However, antidepressants alone may help alleviate anxiety symptoms, especially the SSRIs.

In the past, doctors usually prescribed barbiturates for anxiety, but because of their addictive and sedating effects, other drugs were developed. Today, most doctors usually prescribe either a drug in the class of medications known as benzodiazepines or a separate drug called busprion. They work in slightly different ways to help calm and relax the anxious person and to remove the troubling symptoms of rapid heartbeat, difficulty with concentration, irritability, stomachaches, and breathing problems. Please note: If you are taking birth control pills, let your doctor know. The estrogen in the Pill may reduce the effects of antianxiety drugs while increasing their side effects.

Benzodiazepines

Although highly effective in relieving anxiety symptoms, benzodiazepines can be addictive if taken for more than a few weeks. Benzodiazepines differ in duration of action in different individuals. They may be taken two or three times a day, or sometimes only once a day. The dosage is usually started at a low level and gradually raised until symptoms are diminished or removed.

General side effects: Benzodiazepines have few side effects, and most that do occur tend to be mild and disappear on their own within a few weeks. In some people, they cause drowsiness and mental slowing or confusion (which is why you shouldn't drive or operate heavy machinery until you know how you are affected by the medication). It is wise not to drink alcohol when taking benzodiazepines, as an interaction between the two can cause life-threatening complications. Be sure to consult with your doctor before discontinuing a benzodiazepine; a withdrawal reaction may occur if you abruptly stop. Withdrawal reactions are similar to anxiety symptoms themselves—shakiness, dizziness, sleeplessness—and thus may be mistaken for a return of anxiety. Your doctor will help you taper your dosage until you can safely stop taking the drug altogether.

ALPRAZOLAM (XANAX)

Dosage: .25 to 1.5 mg per day up to 6 to 8 mg per day.
Special Considerations: Alprazolam is known to relieve anxiety symptoms very quickly, sometimes within a day or two of taking the first dose, usually within a week. For depressive symptoms or for panic disorder, it may take two to three weeks for its full effects to take hold. Alprazolam can be highly addictive, and withdrawal is difficult. The drug should gradually be tapered off to minimize withdrawal symptoms.

LORAZEPAN (ATIVAN)

Dosage: 2 to 6 mg per day divided into smaller doses.
Special considerations: It is especially important to check with your doctor before combining Ativan with barbiturates or any sedative-type medication. Do not discontinue Ativan without first discussing it with your doctor; you may experience withdrawal symptoms if you stop using it abruptly.

CLONAZEPAM (KLONOPIN)

Dosage: 1.5 mg per day up to a usual maximum of 8 to 10 mg per day.

Special Considerations: Klonopin also works very quickly to relieve anxiety symptoms, and may also help to improve concentration and symptoms of lethargy that may accompany a coexisting depression. Klonopin may be addictive.

DIAZEPAM (VALIUM)

Dosage: 2 to 5 mg per day up to a maximum of 40 mg per day.

Special Considerations: Once one of the most widely prescribed psychotherapeutic drugs, Valium has been largely supplanted by other drugs, like those listed above, that are less psychologically and physically addictive.

Buspirone (BuSpar)

Buspirone belongs to a family of medications called *azaspirones* and works to relieve anxiety by increasing serotonin activity in the brain. It is used primarily for treatment of generalized anxiety disorder, and is especially useful in treating anxiety associated with depressive symptoms.

Dosage: 10 to 15 mg per day divided into two or three doses, with increases up to a maximum dose of 60 mg per day.

Special Considerations: Side effects, including dizziness, dry mouth, diarrhea, headache, nausea, and nervousness, are usually short-lived and mild. Buspirone tends to be slower acting than the benzodiazepines, so it may take almost a month to reap its full benefits.

Questions and Answers about Medication Management

Many if not most women who take antidepressants find the process relatively easy and problem-free, especially after the first few weeks when the drugs "kick in" to improve symptoms and most side effects have abated. Nevertheless, you'll no doubt have questions, now or as your therapy continues about the drugs you're taking and how they are supposed to work. Please discuss your concerns with your doctor. In the meantime, here are some of the most commonly asked questions about antidepressant drug therapy.

▼ *How quickly will symptoms go away?*

Although you might experience some improvement—such as increased energy—within a week, it's more likely that you won't feel much of a change in mood for three to four weeks. If you need to increase your dose or try a different medication, it might take another few weeks for improvement to occur, and even longer before you feel the medication's full impact.

▼ *What happens if the medication doesn't work, or if it causes unpleasant side effects?*

Taking medication of any kind requires a certain amount of responsibility on your part. It's up to you to tell your doctor how the medication seems to be working and what side effects (if any) they cause.

The important thing is not to get discouraged: Many people need to try a few different dosages, different drugs, or even a combination of medications before hitting upon the right solution for them. Fortunately, more than 65 percent of people who do not respond to one type of drug will improve on another.

If you do not respond at all to the chosen medication or

if you experience side effects that do not subside, your doctor may decide to: (1) change the dosage, (2) try a different drug in the same class of antidepressants, (3) switch you to a drug from a different class, or (4) try a combination of medications. If you only feel a little better on a particular medication, your doctor might decide to augment your therapy with the addition of another type of drug, such as thyroid supplements or stimulants. A short course of stimulants, for instance, may help improve stubborn symptoms of fatigue and listlessness.

If your condition fails to improve, and you are seriously depressed, your doctor may suggest electroconvulsive therapy (ECT). You'll find more information about ECT later in the chapter.

▼ *What happens if my doctor switches me from one medication to another? Do I have to wait in between?*

In some cases, you can make the transition immediately. In others, you'll have to observe what doctors call a "washout" period to get one drug out of your system before introducing another. When switching from an MAOI to a TCA or SSRI, doctors usually recommend a two-week or longer wait depending upon the specific drug chosen. Be sure to follow your doctor's instructions.

▼ *Besides switching medications, are there other ways to alleviate side effects?*

In chapter 7, we provide you with lots of tips about coping with both relatively mild side effects and more serious concerns. If you find a drug that alleviates your depressive symptoms successfully, but causes particularly unpleasant and stubborn side effects, your doctor may decide to add a drug to alleviate the side effects instead of looking for another antidepressant.

▼ *How long will I have to take medication?*

That's an issue for you and your doctor to decide together based on your current condition and how fast you improve. As a general rule, once you've been symptom-free for about six months, you and your doctor might decide to taper your medication dose while carefully watching for the recurrence of symptoms.

If symptoms do recur, or if you have had recurrent depressive episodes in the past, you may require long-term drug therapy in order to stay well. Fortunately, we know that long-term use of most antidepressants is safe: Some women have taken antidepressants for as long as thirty years with no ill effects.

▼ *Can I drink alcohol while taking antidepressants?*

Most doctors strongly discourage using alcohol while on medication. Not only does alcohol depress the central nervous system, but it stimulates enzymes that break down the medication, lowering the amount in the blood and thus making it more difficult to maintain therapeutic levels. Alcohol also tends to enhance the sedating effects of antidepressants that cause drowsiness as an initial side effect.

▼ *If I'm having a particularly bad day, would it be okay to take more medication?*

Generally speaking, it is unwise for you to alter the dosage of any medication you take unless you have your doctor's explicit instructions to do so. Ask your doctor what to do under various circumstances: if you have a bad day, if you forget to take your medication, if you take more than the suggested dose, etc. That way, you'll be less likely to suffer any adverse reactions should you take more or less medication than usual.

▼ *If I take a medication that works for me, will my depression disappear?*

It's important for you to understand the limits of medication. Although antidepressants can dramatically change the way you feel, you may well face other challenges—challenges that drug therapy will not automatically allow you to meet. Depending on how severe and long-standing your depression has been, you may be suffering from low self-esteem, you may have learned nonproductive thought and behavior patterns to compensate for your blue moods and low energy, and/or have relationships that are in need of some repair. See chapter 6 for more information about how psychotherapy can help you sort out your priorities and start on your path to a fuller life.

A WORD ABOUT
ELECTROCONVULSIVE
THERAPY (ECT)

Formerly known as "shock therapy," ECT is the treatment of choice for individuals with severe depression who are suicidal, delusional, or whose disorder is life-threatening. The National Institute of Mental Health estimates that about 110,000 people each year receive ECT.

Marjorie and her son, Robert, discussed ECT with Marjorie's doctor before deciding it was necessary to alleviate her suicidal tendencies.

"I wanted to die," Marjorie remembers. "ECT scared me, but anything was better than feeling like I did. It felt a little strange, and I had trouble remembering things for a while after the treatment, but it really did snap me out of it."

Scientists are unsure as to how and why ECT works to alleviate depressive symptoms. They believe that it may alter receptors for the same group of neurotransmitters that tricyclic antidepressants affect, and they know it temporarily shuts down certain nerve pathways in the brain. Beyond that, however, they just don't know.

Although the general public still harbors fearsome images of ECT—some of them promulgated by the excellent but outdated movie *One Flew Over the Cuckoo's Nest*—ECT is a simple and painless procedure. If you decide to undergo ECT, your doctor will place you under general anesthesia as well as give you a muscle relaxant to minimize muscular response during the treatment. Usually patients receive about eight to twelve treatments over a three-week period, but your doctor will provide a regimen appropriate for you based on your individual needs.

With ECT, you'll probably feel a little confused and perhaps agitated for a short period after each treatment. It is also likely that you'll experience what is called *retrograde amnesia:* a failure to recall events that occurred within a few months before and after the treatment. You may also find your ability to learn and retain new information is hampered for several weeks. In all but 1 in 200 patients (as estimated by the American Psychiatric Association), memory returns to normal and memories of past events are recovered.

Who Should Have ECT?

In addition to people like Marjorie who suffer from psychotic and/or suicidal depression, other individuals who might benefit from ECT are women who:

▼ Do not improve with either medication, psychotherapy, or a combination
▼ Cannot tolerate side effects of psychiatric medication (often because of their advanced age or because they are pregnant)
▼ Have a medical condition for which antidepressants are dangerous
▼ Have improved with ECT in the past

Who Should Avoid ECT?

There are a number of people whose medical conditions would put them at risk for serious complications with ECT. These include women who have:

▼ Angina or a recent heart attack
▼ Aneurysms in the brain or aorta
▼ Severe hypertension

You've now received an overview of the medical options, including medication and ECT, available to treat your depression. In most cases of depression, these options will succeed only if you combine them with psychotherapy, which we discuss in depth in chapter 6.

6
▼
THERAPY FOR WOMEN, COUPLES, AND FAMILIES

In chapter 5, we explored the potential of antidepressants and other psychotherapeutic drugs to help those with depression break free of their illness. It is true that medication is often an integral part of therapy for depression, anxiety, and related disorders. For many people, it represents the best hope for a return to relatively stable mental state. It is rare, however, that psychotherapeutic drugs alone can solve the whole spectrum of symptoms and side effects—physical, emotional, and practical—that depression can cause.

If you're like most women who have suffered through depression, you need more than medication to navigate through your current situation and the next stage of your life. For one thing, you may still harbor guilt or confusion over mistakes you feel you made while depressed, or you may continue to contend with feelings of low self-esteem. You may feel too paralyzed to make any decisions, even about treatment. You also may need help in identifying the sources of stress that helped to trigger the depression in the first place, and then guidance in developing more positive ways to cope. This process is often a painful and difficult one.

"For me, medication was a double-edged sword," Marilyn admits. My eating disorder allowed me to stuff my emotions—about myself, about my parents, about school—so far down I couldn't feel them anymore. I didn't even know they were there. The medication allowed me to connect again. It felt good, but it was also painful and a little scary. It was like looking at the past through a different lens, one with a clearer focus. I need therapy to help me through this, there's no doubt about it."

Julia's challenges were more practical in nature. "I realized I'd lived most of my life undermining myself every step of the way, with my drinking and in my relationships. I wanted therapy not only to help me feel better now, but also to help me avoid falling into those same traps again."

Past mistakes, current complications, future goals—for many women, especially those coping with depression, psychotherapy helps put them all into proper perspective. What about you? Do you feel you could benefit from seeing a professional trained to help you sort through your emotions, better understand your behavior, and set some realistic goals for your future?

In this chapter, we offer tips on identifying what you should expect from therapy, finding a qualified mental health professional, and establishing a successful partnership with your therapist. First, though, let's take a look at what therapy can do to help someone suffering with depression.

DEFINING THE GOALS OF THERAPY

As you'll see later in the chapter, many types of psycho-therapy exist, each one addressing issues and concerns in a slightly different way. In the end, however, they all have the same ultimate objective: to help you reestablish connections with your full range of emotions—joy as well as sadness, pride as well as shame and guilt, strength as well as fear, anticipation as well as disappointment—and to look at the world and your position with more objectivity, optimism, and energy.

Here are just some of the goals of therapy you should consider for yourself.

Feeling Better

You should aim to alleviate your symptoms of depression first, before you attempt to address any deeper or more complicated issues. Simply getting yourself to a therapist may well make you feel as if you've gained some positive control over your situation. For many people, medication is the quickest way to feel better. Other strategies, which we discuss in further depth in chapter 7, involve getting some exercise and reestablishing regular eating and sleeping habits as much as possible. These keys to physical well-being contribute more than you might realize to the state of your mental health.

Identifying Sources of Stress or Unhappiness

Once you've regained some of your energy and powers of concentration, you and your therapist can begin to look at what has triggered the depression in the first place. Did you lose a job recently? Did a relationship you value end? Do you have unresolved feelings of guilt or anger in a particular relationship? Are you not living up to your own expectations? Is there another aspect of your life that is causing you stress? These factors might be obvious to you or they may be hidden beneath layers of self-doubt and confusion.

Making an Accurate Appraisal of Your Current Situation

It probably seems to you as if your life is out of control and unmanageable. Maybe you think you've damaged some of your relationships beyond repair. A therapist will help you to more objectively assess what in your life needs fixing, and what is more on track than you think.

Identifying and Changing Self-defeating Thought Patterns and Behaviors

If you're like most people who suffer from depression, you've made a kind of internal audiotape of self-criticism and pessimistic thoughts. You play it back every time you try to start to enjoy a favorite hobby or begin a new project or make a vow to get back into the social swing of things. The tape might say, "You were never good at knitting anyway, why bother?" or "Remember the last time you made a proposal to your boss? He turned you down flat," or "What's the point in going to the party? I never have a good time anyway."

One of the most important goals of therapy is to erase this tape and make a new one filled with more positive, self-affirming thoughts. Recent research suggests that optimism is an underrated ally in the battle against depression. In fact, a positive mental outlook helps slow the aging process; optimists actually live longer, on average, than do pessimists. That's one reason the flagship journal of the American Psychological Association began the year 2000 with a special issue devoted to "positive psychology."

Learning to Set Realistic Goals

As you become more depressed, your goals seem to become more and more impossible to attain. If you're like most people in the midst of a depression, your life right now looks out of control. You feel overwhelmed by the laundry piled up in the closet, the unpaid bills stuffed in the kitchen drawer, and the tough work assignments languishing half done at the office. A therapist can help you set priorities and break down larger tasks into smaller more manageable ones until, slowly but surely, you reduce what currently might seem like a mountain of unmet obligations.

Rebuilding Self-esteem

One of the most damaging aspects of depression is the way it can undermine your confidence and feelings of self-worth. Therapy can help you identify your strengths and minimize your weaknesses, while helping you to see that you're still a worthwhile person.

Identifying Sources of Support and
Learning How to Ask for Help

As discussed in chapter 1, depression is one of the most
isolating of all chronic illnesses. It's likely that you've shut
yourself off from friends and loved ones as you've struggled, alone, with your feelings. With help from your therapist, you can identify the people in your life you most want
to connect with again, and learn to ask for their support in
direct, appropriate ways.

CHOOSING A THERAPIST

As you may remember from chapter 2, there are several
different types of mental health professionals who can
help you work through your depression and toward the
goals we discussed above. Most likely you'll choose either a
psychiatrist (a medical doctor with special training in mental health), a psychologist (someone with a doctoral degree in psychology and clinical experience in treating mental
and emotional illness), or a social worker who specializes
in psychotherapy. Psychiatric nurses, pastoral counselors,
alcohol counselors, and other types of therapists are also
available.

How should you decide what type of therapist to
choose? And what individual among that group might be
right for you? These days, it's probably wise to start by
checking with your medical insurance or health plan to
see if it covers mental health services and, if so, how you
may obtain these benefits. Many policies have arbitrary
limits and may only cover 50 percent of the costs of a fixed
number of visits per year. If you're one of the increasing
numbers of Americans who is a member of a health maintenance organization, for instance, you may be limited in

your freedom to choose who can treat you and how long you are to be treated.

You may use your HMO or managed care plan or you may want to seek care outside with your own funds if you are able. The advantage of paying for care yourself is that you will not have restrictions on how many sessions you may have or what therapist you may choose to visit. Most therapists of all types see people in private practice ouside of HMOs. They will usually accept insurance as payment or part payment and make a fee arrangement with you.

"I had a very frustrating experience with my HMO," Jordan describes. "Normally, I'm quite thrilled with their services. I love my gynecologist, for instance, and see her on a regular basis. But when it came to getting help for my depression, it was a little confusing. It took about three weeks to get the first appointment with a licensed social worker. He was very nice and supportive, and helped me start thinking about my problems. But then I needed to wait another week before I could see a psychiatrist for a prescription for antidepressants. My HMO only covered sixteen visits a year, and because of scheduling problems, I could only see my therapist once every two or three weeks. I know if I were suicidal or very ill, the HMO would cover everything, but I couldn't get what I really wanted—a regular weekly appointment with a therapist."

Once you know from what pool of therapists you can draw, you might want to ask your primary care physician to recommend who among them might be right for you. Ask for a couple of suggestions, as well as a copy of your medical records so that the therapist has them to examine at your first appointment.

If you need further referrals, your local medical or psychiatric society (see Resources), community mental health center, and medical school are also good sources. You should feel free to specify a therapist's age, sex, race, or religious background, if any of those factors are important to you. (In this book, we use the pronoun "she" because this is a book by and for women but there obviously are many excellent male therapists skilled at treating women with depression.) Other medical and psychiatric societies can tell you where psychiatrists went to school, took residency training, and whether they are certified by the American Board of Psychiatry and Neurology.

Select two or three therapists and phone for information about appointment availability, location, and cost of the first visit. At your first appointment, ask questions about fees, appointment flexibility, cancellation policy, and insurance form procedures or HMO co-payment policies. Most important, ask the therapist how much experience she has in treating depression, what kinds of approaches she feels most comfortable using (we discuss those approaches later in the chapter), and how many sessions she usually suggests to treat depression.

After your initial session, think about how you felt with the therapist. Did you feel she listened to you and had a sense of your pain and your problems? Did you trust her? Did you feel relatively at ease talking to her about your problems? Only if you believe you can establish a trusting, comfortable relationship (called the *therapeutic alliance*)—one that allows you to reveal your innermost feelings to an accepting and supportive professional—should you agree to continue with the therapist. Do keep in mind that it may take time for such a solid relationship to develop, but you should feel from the start that the potential exists. Please note that if you feel uncomfortable or dissatisfied with either the relationship or your progress at any point during therapy, you should not hesitate to talk to the therapist about it and even to change therapists.

Once you choose a therapist you think might work for you, you're ready to start the hard but rewarding work of sorting through the emotional and practical problems underlying and complicating your depression. There are several different ways to approach this task, and we describe them here.

Understanding Therapeutic Approaches

Most mental health professionals today are trained in a variety of psychotherapeutic techniques. The person you choose will probably tailor his or her approach to your particular problem, personality, and needs. She will make a careful assessment of your current problem, including the circumstances that led to your depression, and your past psychological history, family history, and medical history. She will then recommend a course of treatment appropriate for you. It may involve some combination of individual, family, and group therapy as well as medication.

If you start with individual therapy (and you most probably will), it may include one or a combination of the following.

INDIVIDUAL THERAPY

Psychodynamic Psychotherapy

Psychodynamic therapy is based on the premise that current difficulties are often the result of unresolved past conflicts. By bringing these conflicts into present awareness, the patient can understand and deal with them in a more appropriate manner. If your therapist chooses this approach, she'll encourage you to talk about past experiences and see what impact they might have on your current situation. The therapist will act as a guide to building greater self-awareness and understanding. This will allow you to gain some measure of control over your life and, hopefully, to make more positive choices in the future.

A popular type of psychodynamic psychotherapy, called *brief dynamic psychotherapy*, concentrates on only those issues directly related to your depression. For instance, if you believe that your symptoms stem from a recent loss of a job, the therapist will help you address both your feelings about the loss as well as the practical and financial aspects that are making it difficult for you to cope.

"My therapist got me to see how much trouble I was having—and it was way more trouble than I realized—making the transition from student to so-called adult," Phoebe relates. "She helped me to work out some options and priorities, and by doing that, gave me a better perspective on what was going on. It didn't happen overnight, but I did eventually feel much less panicked and stuck."

Psychodynamic psychotherapy may be brief, consisting of less than twenty-five weekly sessions, or long-term, with one or two sessions a week over a period of several years. Some people with chronic depression may find psychodynamic psychotherapy helpful in resolving long-standing issues, thought patterns, and behaviors.

Cognitive Behavorial Therapy

"I know I've gotten myself into a vicious cycle sort of trap in my thinking," admits Jordan. "I'll start out feeling positive, or at least neutral about a writing assignment. I'll do the research for the article, enjoy the planning, but then, as soon as something goes wrong—if I can't get started on the writing or if a few pages turn out clumsy—I'll tell myself 'Who are you kidding, you're no writer. And if you turn this in, everyone will know the truth.' Well, I don't really use those words exactly, it's only because I've been in therapy for a while that I see that I'm doing it, but those negative thoughts are always there. No wonder I haven't been able to work as well as I'd like."

Jordan and her therapist are attacking Jordan's professional difficulties using a psychotherapeutic method called cognitive behavioral therapy. What's behind this type of therapy is the idea that self-criticism and negative thinking patterns can trigger depression. In other words, it could be that your view of yourself and your place in the world control or direct your emotions. If you constantly berate yourself, expect yourself to fail, and make negative (usually inaccurate) assessments of what others think of you, depression is sure to be the end result.

If you and your therapist decide to try cognitive behavioral therapy, you'll work to reframe these negative thought patterns, to change them into realistic and reaffirming ones. You'll learn to become more aware of the thoughts and attitudes that depress you, to challenge their validity, and then to replace them with more positive alternatives.

The first step in this approach involves identifying the specific types of negative thoughts you harbor. Which among these dysfunctional thinking patterns do you follow?

ALL-OR-NOTHING THINKING

Do you think only in extremes? If you gain two pounds one week do you see yourself as a fat slob with no will power? If your boss rejects one of your ideas, do you conclude you're a failure with no chance of ever getting ahead?

MAGNIFYING OR MINIMIZING

If you stub your toe getting out of bed in the morning, do you automatically conclude that your day is sure to be a bad one? If your husband pays you a compliment, do you assume it's because he wants something or must have done something he feels guilty about?

OVERGENERALIZATION

If you fail one course in college, do you conclude that you're stupid and unable to learn anything? Do you leap to a long-range conclusion based on one event? If a date stands you up, for instance, do you think that you'll never go out again? If you miss a deadline at work, do you assume you'll be fired or never asked to participate in a project again?

PERSONALIZATION

How often do you relate a negative event—one that has nothing to do with you—to something about you or the way you behave? If someone shoves you while getting onto the subway, do you lay the blame on his shoulders for being rude, or do you assume you were in the way, or too fat, or not quick enough to move out of his path?

AUTOMATIC THOUGHTS

If your first thoughts whenever you attempt to throw a dinner party or start a new eating or exercise plan are "It'll never work out" and "I know I'll screw up," you're taking part in automatic thinking that's sure to undermine your efforts.

Once you figure out what kinds of undermining thought patterns you've created, your therapist will help you to restructure the patterns and refocus your behavior. One specific cognitive therapy is called "cognitive rehearsal." Here, you envision a challenging or troubling situation, imagine how you might meet or solve it, then break the process down into manageable steps. With help from your therapist, you'd rehearse each step mentally, erasing the negative thoughts—the "I can'ts"—and replace them with "I will" and "I can." Other methods involve keeping a diary of activities, reviewing it with your therapist, and then receiving instructions for addressing problems with your social or practical life. For instance, if you've withdrawn from your friends, your therapist might help you schedule some time for phone calls or coffee breaks with people during the week. You'll be asked to keep those dates as if they were business appointments, even if you feel negatively about them.

"I hadn't been shopping with my daughter for more than two months," Beth confesses. "It was all I could do to go. But it was an 'assignment,' so I did it. And you know what? Once I got there, it was all right. Pleasant, really. I only wish Sandy hadn't been so uncomfortable with me. I guess we'll work through that eventually."

Cognitive behavioral therapy is relatively brief (usually sixteen to twenty sessions) and works to address your most pressing concerns. A related type of psychotherapy is called behavioral therapy.

Behavioral Therapy

As its name implies, behavioral therapy concentrates on identifying and changing negative patterns of behavior, rather than thought patterns, as is true for cognitive behavior therapy. Behavioral therapy is especially helpful for disorders characterized by specific abnormal ways of acting, such as substance abuse, alcoholism, or eating disorders. It tends to be less helpful than interpersonal or cognitive behavioral therapy in treating major depression, but may be useful if you also suffer from bulimia or an anxiety disorder.

If you decide to participate in behavioral therapy, the therapist will give you "homework assignments"—specific tasks you must accomplish by the next therapy session— encourage you to succeed, and monitor your progress. There are several techniques that she might use to help you change your negative patterns into more positive ones.

▼ *Behavior modification* attempts to reward good behavior while discouraging negative habits in an effort to break undermining patterns. Your therapist might encourage you to treat yourself to a manicure (or another pleasurable activity), for instance, every time you manage to keep a date with a friend or finish an assignment at work on time.

▼ *Systematic desensitization and exposure therapy* are two successful methods of dealing with anxiety or phobias that, as discussed, often occur in combination with depression. They help you learn to control or reduce fear triggered by specific situations or objects by exposing you to them bit by bit over time. Gail, who's become agoraphobic and finds it difficult to go outside with her son, gradually learned to leave the house by first looking at photographs of mothers and children playing in the park, then going outside in the yard for just a few minutes alone, then taking her son for a short walk, and so on.

"It took a while," Gail remembers, "and I have to admit, I felt a little idiotic, but it was much better than that horrible panic I used to feel whenever I'd even think about opening the door and walking outside."

Interpersonal Psychotherapy

According to studies conducted by the National Institute of Mental Health, interpersonal therapy is one of the most promising types of individual therapy when it comes to treating depression. Interpersonal psychotherapy (IPT) is usually fairly short term—it normally consists of twelve to sixteen weekly sessions—and focuses on correcting current problems in your life. This therapy is based on the theory that disturbed social and personal relationships can cause or precipitate depression. In turn, the illness may make these relationships or situations more problematic. The therapist helps the patient understand how depression and interpersonal conflicts are related.

Unlike psychoanalytic psychotherapy (discussed briefly below), IPT does not spend a lot of time addressing unconscious phenomena, such as defense mechanisms or internal conflicts. Instead IPT focuses primarily on the "here and now" factors that directly interfere with your ability to cope with the practical, social, and emotional circumstances of your life.

Psychoanalysis

Established by Sigmund Freud in the early part of the twentieth century, psychoanalysis is based on the concept that depression and other mental and emotional disturbances are the result of past conflicts that people push into their unconscious. In very general terms, psychoanalysts work with patients to explore past hurts, failures, and traumas that fester within and prevent patients from living full and satisfying lives.

In most instances, psychoanalysis is not the treatment of choice for people with depression whose mental and emotional problems tend to be—at least to start—more situational and immediate in nature. The process tends to be quite a lengthy and intense one. If you decide to undergo analysis, you'll meet with a psychiatrist at least three to five times a week for at least two years. Some common psychoanalytic techniques include *free association*, in which you speak openly and freely about whatever comes to mind while the analyst remains neutral and relatively passive, and *dream analysis*, in which the analyst attempts to uncover your subconscious desires and fears as they are revealed in the dreams you remember and relate to her.

Although some psychoanalysts today prescribe medication as part of the therapy, especially for their depressed patients, most traditional psychoanalysts do not. The primary therapeutic tool is the relationship that forms between the analyst and patient during the intense and lengthy sessions.

In addition, psychoanalysts may use free association as a way to connect you to any unresolved conflicts from your childhood that have created and perpetuated undermining patterns of behavior and thinking. One thing the analyst looks for are defense mechanisms, or distorted ways of thinking about a situation that interfere with your mental and emotional health. Included among the many defense mechanisms are the following.

▼ *Repression* involves the "stuffing down" of threatening thoughts, impulses, memories, or wishes so that they remain embedded in the unconscious. Peri, for instance, repressed memories of the abuse she suffered at the hands of her grandfather until she was in her early forties and about to start an important relationship.

▼ *Denial*, or the inability to accept a painful or unpleasant reality, is often a natural step in the grief or transition process, but may become problematic if it persists for too long. "I denied my marriage was over for the longest time," Beth remembers. "I mean, literally for years after the divorce was final, I imagined Tony and I would get back together. I never thought of myself as single, even after he got remarried. I didn't realize how much this was hurting me, but now I know that instead of getting on with my life, my denial left me feeling betrayed, abandoned, and lonely much longer than I should have."

▼ *Rationalization* is a way of substituting acceptable reasons for your real motivations. When Gail sits herself in front of the television every night, numbing herself by eating and staring, she convinces herself that she's just "relaxing" after a tough day.

▼ *Intellectualization* allows you to objectify painful feelings or situations so that they do not touch you emotionally but exist only as a kind of intellectual exercise. "Now that I know what the term means, I certainly intellectualized my ex-husband's affair," Beth admits. "For maybe six months after I found out about it, I didn't let myself feel hurt. I just thought about it as if it were someone else's life, or a tragic Russian novel. And I'd dissect my marriage and my husband's motivations endlessly. But I didn't cry. Not for a long time."

There are several other defense mechanisms, all used for the same reason: to keep us from coming to terms with very real, but very painful realities in our pasts and presents. Once your defense mechanisms are identified, your therapist will help you replace them with more helpful and positive coping strategies. These include, among others, the following.

▼ *Sublimation* involves taking an unhealthy impulse and redirecting it toward a more positive and acceptable behavior. Instead of watching television (which she did enjoy) and eating, Gail decided to take up knitting, a hobby that once gave her pleasure. "Now even if I do watch too much television at night"—she smiles—"I have something to show for it—a sweater for my husband or son—at the end of a couple of weeks. That may be rationalization, too, but it *is* actually quite relaxing."

▼ *Humor* helps you to cope by focusing on the ridiculous and comic aspects of life, even the most painful of situations. "I discovered that my sense of humor was the only thing that kept me from ending it all," Gail remarks. "Of course, I didn't find it funny while I was in the middle of it, but as I worked through some stuff, I got to the point where I could laugh at the image of my standing at the doorway—my ordinary little doorway leading to my sweet little front yard—shaking like a leaf, sure that the big bad wolf was ready to pounce. That image got me through the worst parts of the exposure therapy."

▼ *Mastery and control,* the ultimate signs of mental health and maturity, involve the ability to confront a difficult and painful challenge directly and without becoming overwhelmed by either your feelings or the practical aspects it entails.

FAMILY AND MARRIAGE THERAPY

Unlike individual therapy, family therapy and marriage therapy focus not on you as an individual but you as a member of a marital or family unit. Although family and/or marriage therapy is usually not the first choice for women suffering with depression, it can be combined with individual therapy under certain circumstances. If your depression appears to be seriously jeopardizing your marriage, interfering with the family dynamic, or, conversely, if you feel your marriage or family relationships are triggering your feelings of hopelessness and anxiety, then you and your therapist might decide to bring in your husband and/or family to work through these issues.

Depending on the particular problems and relationships in question, your therapist will help you and your family look at the ways your feelings or behavior impacts on those of other members. This therapeutic method is called *systems orientation* because it looks at the family as a unit that works (or fails to work) together. Some of the theories involved in system orientation include:

▼ *Context:* As you probably have discovered already, your struggle with depression probably affects your husband, children, or close family or friends. In turn, their reactions may create more stress and anxiety for you, which could well exacerbate your disease. A therapist can help you identify the pattern of these interactions and see if there are better ways to manage them.

▼ *Interaction:* The way you and your family communicate with one another is just as important as the content of what you say and do. In family therapy, you can learn new and more satisfying ways of relating to one another.

▼ *Fit:* What is "normal" in one family isn't necessarily so in another, as Phoebe found out when she moved in with her boyfriend, Stu. "I was brought up in a pretty loud and raucous family—I had two brothers and two sisters—and so I'm used to arguing and yelling and . . . well, showing my emotions," Phoebe says. "Stu, though, is much more quiet and reserved. I felt a little stifled with him. There was so much he didn't say or express, I kind of held back, too, and I'm just figuring out now how much more stress that put on me. I think we can work this out, though, now that we see what's going on."

▼ *Adaptability:* Are you and your family—as a unit—able to "go with the flow" of changing circumstances? Or is your household either too disorganized and chaotic or too rigid and inflexible to adapt quickly and smoothly? A therapist can help your family develop more effective strategies for facing challenges together and separately so that the overall stress level is lower.

▼ *Cohesion:* Cohesion refers to the relative connectedness and separateness in a couple or family. Does each member of your family tend to act independently and thus find it difficult to come together as a unit to face a crisis like your depression? Family therapy can help your family to acknowledge your interdependence, provide mutual support to one another, and work cooperatively to reach individual and family goals.

GROUP THERAPY AND SELF-HELP ORGANIZATIONS

Group therapy, the most widely used form of psychotherapy today, works toward the same general goals as individual therapy: developing a greater understanding and acceptance of yourself and learning more effective and appropriate coping strategies. As its name suggests, though, the process takes place in a group setting, usually among people with similar problems and life circumstances. The therapist is there to set ground rules, guide discussions, and resolve conflicts, but the bulk of the work is performed by members of the group: By interacting with one another, members can begin to identify patterns of their behavior and personality that may be interfering with healthy relationships outside the group. They challenge one another's defense mechanisms, share insights into common problems, and provide support and empathy within a safe and structured environment.

Group therapy, as well as its lay counterpart, the self-help group, is not usually recommended for someone with depression, at least not at the beginning of therapy when feelings of low self-esteem and low energy need more immediate and one-on-one attention. However, if you have a coexisting substance abuse problem or eating disorder, group therapy can be an excellent way to explore your behaviors and come to terms with the feelings they evoke in you.

You've now had a chance to see the many different strategies used to treat depression and other disorders within a therapeutic setting. In chapter 7, we look at ways you can use these methods of understanding and coping in your own day-to-day life. "Facing the Future with Optimism" shows you how to direct your new-found energy and insight into making your life—at home, at work, and inside your soul—better and more promising today and tomorrow.

IMPORTANT QUESTIONS AND ANSWERS ABOUT CHAPTER 6

Q. I'm a little confused about all the different types of therapy available. I'm thirty-four and suffering with a combination of depression and anxiety. Which type of therapy is best for me?

A. It's impossible to say without knowing a lot more about

you. But don't worry too much about choosing an approach before picking a therapist. As discussed, most therapists use a combination of approaches depending on your symptoms, your personality, and your needs. Then, if one method doesn't work, the therapist will try another, or a variety of others, until you feel better and can cope with your challenges in more effective and healthy ways.

Q. I'm a Hispanic woman from Haiti. Although I'm accustomed to American culture, I come from a different backround and religion, and so look at the world in a different way. Is it important for me to visit a Hispanic therapist?

A. Not necessarily, but you might want to look for someone who's familiar with your heritage or willing to learn something about it as he or she treats you. In November 1995, the *American Journal of Psychiatry* published guidelines for psychiatric evaluation that for the first time explicitly recommended that a therapist consider a patient's cultural or ethnic background, including how the patient understands the illness.

There are some well-recognized disorders of the mind, for instance, that do not exist in all cultures. Anorexia nervosa, for instance, appears to exist in modern industrialized societies like those of the United States and Western Europe but not in Native American or cultures in deveoping countries. In Japan, mental health professionals recognize a malady known as *taijin kyofuso* or "fear of people." A person suffering from taijin kyofuso has a morbid dread of doing something that will embarrass other people and, medical anthropologists believe, revolves around social shame that simply has no equivalent here in the United States.

As multicultural diversity continues to be the rule in

cities and towns, more and more health professionals will be aware of, and able to adapt therapy to, each patient's background. Many teaching institutions across the country now offer students of psychology and psychiatry training on different cultural groups and how to assess the cultural impact on their patients' problems.

Q. If depression is biochemical in origin, why does psychotherapy work to alleviate symptoms?

A. For a number of reasons. First, psychotherapy helps someone make a realistic assessment of her problems, allowing her to see, perhaps for the first time, the ways that depression has undermined her personal, social, and professional life. She'll also learn ways to cope better with the challenges she faces.

Second, as we tried to emphasize in chapter 3, the mind (our emotions and thought processes) and the brain (the tissue and chemicals) are intimately linked. The way we think influences our body and brain chemistry. A study reported in the February 1996 issue of the *Archives of General Psychiatry* described an experiment that used PET (positron emission tomography) scans—sophisticated imaging technology—to show how behavioral therapy can have biological effects. Scientists studied nine people suffering from obsessive-compulsive disorder, an anxiety disorder that compels people to perform certain unproductive acts over and over again. In these people, three parts of the brain that usually act independently become hyperactive together. After undergoing ten weeks of cognitive-behavior therapy—without medication—these brain structures were less hyperactive and, most important, worked more independently from one another. As a result, the patients were less plagued by obsessive-compulsive behavior.

Recovery from any emotional disorder requires putting into action a combination of several techniques, often including medication, therapy, and self-help strategies such as the ones we will explore in chapter 7. What all of these techniques have in common is to get you to see life in a more realistic and positive light and help you to go after your ambitions and dreams with confidence.

▼

FACING THE FUTURE WITH OPTIMISM

"'**G**et some exercise,' my sister kept telling me."—Beth laughs—"Sure thing. That made sense right then, when I could barely get out of bed. Exercise. Ha!"

Marilyn's mother encouraged her to "start eating right" while Gloria's daughter urged her to "get out more." No one had to tell Gail that she needed to manage her time better so that she didn't end the day feeling even more overwhelmed than when she started, but her husband often gave her little "pep talks" about it.

"Everyone means well when they give you advice about 'snapping out' of your depression," Gail relates. "I know my husband tried so hard not to nag, or put more pressure on me to get the housework done or start thinking about going back to work part-time. But, because I already was feeling useless and hopeless, everything he said sounded like criticism to me. He made me feel worse when he was only trying to make me feel better."

As Gail so eloquently describes, depression does more to disrupt daily life than most of us realize. Some women find that their relationships suffer as they withdraw more and more into their emptiness. Others must struggle to meet their responsibilities at work and at home. Each personal or professional disappointment only adds to the low self-esteem and feelings of hopelessness that are the hallmarks of depression.

In this chapter, we provide you with some valuable tools that may help you through your recovery period. Combined with medication and therapy, these coping strategies will help you make it through to the other side of your own personal cloud of depression and despair as easily as possible. In the sections that follow, you'll find a variety of suggestions about day-to-day living and future planning.

Please note that these are only suggestions, not prescriptions. One of the keys to recovering from depression is to avoid adding any stress to your already overburdened situation. If looking at this long list of "to do's" feels overwhelming to you, take your time with it. Look at only one or two suggestions each day, or simply check off the ones that appeal to you and ignore the rest.

COPING WITH SYMPTOMS OF DEPRESSION

As we discussed in chapter 2 and as you've seen in the stories of the women you met throughout the book, the symptoms of depression tend to halt a woman in her tracks, keep her from moving forward, and isolate her from the rest of the world. The following suggestions might help make the reentry process a little easier for you.

Lighten Up Your Thinking

▼ *Erase the negative tapes you play inside your head.* Don't allow yourself to say "I can't" or "what's the use" until you evaluate your situation with objectivity. Try to look for the positive aspects of your behavior and of your circumstances. Psychologist Jay Cleve, who wrote a terrific guidebook for coping with symptoms of depression called *Out of the Blues,* refers to the "inner saboteur" that exists inside of each of us—and which comes out in full force during a depression. This saboteur judges and criticizes your behavior, denies you the ability to recognize your accomplishments, and keeps you from proceeding with new plans and activities with any hope or confidence of success. It's important to hear those voices, recognize them as negative, and replace them with more positive, life-affirming ones.

▼ *Avoid making life decisions.* Needless to say, the midst of a depression is no time for you to be making a major career change or moving to a new city or a decision to start or end a relationship. First, your judgement is not the best right now. Your emotional problems keep you from seeing your strengths and true desires with any clarity. Second, making decisions is a stressful activity, one you should—if at all possible—put off until you feel better. Otherwise you risk undermining your progress.

"The last thing I should have ever tried to do was consider my job options," Marjorie admits. "There I was in the midst of a psychotic depression trying to navigate through a maze of politics at work. I can't tell you how close I came to quitting or being fired. I finally got up enough courage to ask my boss—well, actually my boss's boss, who was more understanding and had more authority—for a short leave of absence. Now that the crisis has passed, I can look at what should happen next with more objectivity and realism."

▼ *Be kind to yourself.* Stop finding fault with everything about yourself and start being kind to yourself. Treat yourself to simple pleasures—brew a cup of your favorite tea and sip it outside in the sun, read a trashy romance novel without harboring a trace of guilt about "wasting time," buy yourself some fresh-cut flowers and put some in every room. Treating yourself doesn't have to cost money, or involve abrogating your responsibilities. Simply take the time to applaud a goal you've met, a decision you've made, a good day you've spent, with something that makes you smile.

Structure Your Recovery

▼ *Give yourself time.* If you've already started your medication or psychotherapy, you probably already feel a bit better. But don't let this resurgence of energy fool you. You may not be ready to take on new responbilities, or even assume all of your previous ones.

"I thought, well, I'll just make myself snap out of it." Rebecca admits. "I'll just put a plan of action into effect and everything'll be okay. I took a second job, I found a new babysitter for my daughter, I even started an exercise class. I held it together for about two weeks, and then fell apart again. I had to start all over, in a way. Now I'm taking my time."

You too may want to slow down your recovery process a bit, evaluate your situation carefully, then slowly but surely begin the process of repair and rebuilding. That's why it's especially helpful to work with a therapist who can aid you in recognizing your limitations and assist you in setting realistic goals.

▼ *Learn to set priorities.* Right now, you might very well be overwhelmed by the tasks before you. Depending on how severe and long-standing your depression is, you may have financial problems caused by your withdrawal; your house-keeping skills may have created some organization problems; or your social life may be in serious need of repair. Working with a therapist, or with a trusted friend, figure out what aspects of your life you'd like to tackle first.

▼ *Develop a time-management plan that works for you.* Many people with depression find that adding a layer of structure and continuity to their lives can be extremely helpful. Start by making a list of daily activities. It can be as simple as (1) Make breakfast. (2) Shower. (3) Go for a walk. (4) Call a friend. (5) Make a shopping list for dinner. (6) Go to the store, etc. Once you feel comfortable and more in control, you can make the same list, but put some time limits to each activity so that you can make the most out of your day. Every time you finish a task, cross it off your list; every time you do, your self-esteem will get a healthy little boost.

Open Yourself Up to Others— and to Yourself

▼ *Schedule time to be with the people you love.* If you're like most women with depression, you've shut yourself off from the people in your life. You might have done so because you don't want to burden them with your feelings of unhappiness or despair, or you may simply lack the energy to communicate. Once you start to feel a little better, though, it's important to start bridging any gaps that exist between you and your friends and family.

"I realized that not only was my husband worried about me and my health, he was worried about *us*," Gail recalls.

"When we were first together, we shared everything. When the depression hit, I withdrew completely, both sexually and as his friend. My therapist helped me to see how abandoned and lonely he felt—and still feels to some extent—and how I had to find ways to bring him back into my world. Now I make sure that we share a meal or two every week without the baby, and I even leave him little notes in his briefcase reassuring him of my love. At first, I thought it was kind of stupid, these little things, but it makes both of us feel better and more connected."

Like Gail, start small. Make a coffee date with a good friend, organize a picnic just for you and your husband, rent a movie and watch it with your kids. Work with your therapist on finding ways to heal any relationship breaches.

▼ *Try to identify what makes you happy and find ways to bring those people or activities back into your life.* What often gets lost in depression is what, in your heart of hearts, satisfies you and brings you pleasure. You may have told yourself that your desires are petty or unimportant, or that you simply don't deserve to be happy. This is negative thinking at its most undermining, and will lead only to further feelings of hopelessness and despair. If you love to read fiction, don't tell yourself it's a "waste of time." Instead, join a book group with others who share your passion so that you'll have some support.

▼ *Ask trusted others for positive feedback.* As you begin to set priorities and make plans, it might be helpful for you to have some kind of feedback system set up to monitor your progress and encourage you along the way.

"I got my sister to help me," Beth recalls. "She's always there to pick me up if I fail or think I'm failing. It's not that she's just a cheerleader or a yes person, but she's willing to help me put things into a more positive light whenever possible. When I decided to take a course at the extension school, but then had to drop out because it interfered with time I wanted to spend with my kids, she didn't criticize me. Instead, she let me know that I made a good decision, that my priorities were the right ones for me at the time. It made a big difference—it kept me from telling myself I was too stupid or too lazy or too . . . depressed to succeed!"

Live Well

The clichés are endless: "You are what you eat," and "A healthy body is a healthy mind," to cite just two. In this instance, though, the clichés have important merit: If you don't treat your body with care, your mind and your emotions will undoubtedly suffer. Here are a few tips to help you get your physical life under control:

▼ *Sleep well.* As you may remember from chapter 2, sleep problems are often the first and most serious symptom of depression. Without question, the less sleep you get, and the less regularly you get it, the more likely you are to suffer from mood-related disorders. The key is to establish a regular sleeping schedule. Follow these tips if you have trouble sleeping:

—Exercise regularly. Physical activity both reduces stress and relaxes your muscles. Try not to exercise in the evening, however, when activity may act as a stimulant.

—Try to go to bed and get up at specific, set times every day and night. Most important, get up at the same time every morning, even if you've had a bad night's sleep, and try to stay up until your regular bedtime. Even if you have to drag yourself through one or two days, it's likely you'll eventually synchronize your body clock so that you'll fall asleep when you're tired and get up feeling refreshed.

—Drink a glass of warm milk. Sometimes the oldest cures are also the most effective. If you can't seem to fall asleep, try drinking a glass of warm milk about a half hour before going to bed. Milk includes high dosages of tryptophan, an amino acid that is the precursor of melatonin (the hormone that scientists believe "sets" the body's internal clock).

—Start keeping a diary. Many people with depression find the dark quiet of night the perfect time to brood on their problems and dwell on their shortcomings. If you write down your fears and worries before you go to bed, you may find yourself feeling less stressed and anxious when it's time to sleep.

▼ *Enjoy a healthy diet.* Food is not only nourishment that provides your body with the raw materials it needs to function. It should also be a source of pleasure. Unfortunately, too many people, especially women, are so afraid of food— of its calories, fat content, of the potential carcinogens it harbors—and our response to it that we've lost the ability to enjoy cooking, eating, and sharing meals with others.

If you're one of the many women who avoid dietary fat and cholesterol like the plague, consider a controversial 1999 study linking depression with lower-than-average blood cholesterol levels. When Duke University psychologist Edward Suarez, working with 121 female volunteers, compared the women's psychological-test scores with their blood-test results, he found that those whose blood cholesterol was under 160 milligrams per deciliter were twice as likely to be depressed than were the women whose blood cholesterol was higher. Suarez speculates that without enough cholesterol, the brain doesn't get enough of the feel-good neurotransmitter serotonin.

In addition to learning the basics of a healthy diet, you should strive to take the time to enjoy the sensual aspects of eating. Smell the food as it cooks, feel its textures as you chew, savor its flavors. At least once in a while, plan special meals for you and your family, times when you can enjoy the pleasures of conversation along with your food.

▼ *Avoid alcohol.* As discussed, people prone to depression all too often use alcohol as a form of self-medication, and an ultimately undermining form at that since it acts as a depressant on the central nervous system. While you're depressed, it is probably wise to avoid alcohol altogether. As long as you don't have an addiction to alcohol, you should feel free to enjoy a glass of wine or an occasional drink once you're feeling better, if you like.

▼ *Exercise.* The benefits of physical activity are almost too numerous to mention. In addition to reducing your risk of developing heart disease, high blood pressure, some kinds of cancer, and a myriad of other diseases, exercise can dramatically improve the quality of the life you live today. It allows you to connect with your physical body, while allowing your mind to take a bit of a break. Indeed, many women with depression who exercise claim it is the one time in their day that they feel relief from their symptoms. Part of the reason is that certain brain chemicals called endorphins, known to dull pain and invoke mild euphoria, are released whenever the body feels pain, including during vigorous exercise when the muscles begin to tire and "burn."

It is important to note, however, that exercise need not be demanding or elaborate to be effective: Moderate exercise—defined as thirty minutes of daily light activity (such as walking, gardening, housecleaning)—is almost as beneficial to one's health as higher level of activities (such as jogging or aerobics). The important thing is to set realistic goals and to choose activities you enjoy. If you've been sedentary for a number of months or years, deciding to train for next month's marathon would be counterproductive, both physically (you're liable to hurt yourself) and emotionally (by setting yourself an impossible goal, you're sure to feel like a failure when you don't meet it). Instead, start slowly. Take a walk around your neighborhood. Perform some stretching exercises on the floor while you watch the news or a favorite sitcom. Join a gym that has a pool and enjoy the sensual pleasure of gliding through the cool water.

▼ *Establish an ease with your mind-body connection.* Stress is a fact of life for women living in late-twentieth-century America, and it's a special burden for those of us who also suffer from depression. Although there is no way to avoid stress—in fact, stress can act as an appropriate and energizing stimulus to activity—you can lessen its potentially damaging effects by learning to help your body and mind relax for certain periods of time each day.

We really have two goals when it comes to stress reduction. The short-term goal involves finding ways to alleviate feelings of anxiety when they occur or preventing them from taking hold at all. The long-term goal involves achieving a more permanent sense of balance and confidence in yourself and your goals.

Without question, the short-term goals are easier to achieve. There are any number of ways to de-stress in the short term. They include, among others:

Biofeedback: One of the most scientific ways of exploring and utilizing the mind-body connection, biofeedback was developed when studies showed that animals could control bodily functions once thought to be completely automatic by being given a reward or punishment. Physicians adapted those findings to design ways for humans to control unconscious functions through conscious thought.

Although there are several biofeedback methods, they all have three things in common: (1) they measure a physiological function (such as muscle tension or heart rate); (2) they convert this measurement to an understandable form (like a computer-generated graph or chart, a blinking light, mercury levels in a thermometer, etc.); and (3) they feed this information back to you.

If you have particular problems dealing with stress, talk to your therapist about biofeedback. It might help you to understand the way your thought processes affect your body, and vice versa, in a more tangible way.

Guided Imagery: The human imagination—the part of our hearts and minds that can picture and sense images and feelings—is one of the most potent health resources available to you. By utilizing the power of your mind, you can help evoke a physical and emotional response in your body in order to relax your muscles, stimulate your immune system, and reduce your physical and emotional pain.

"My therapist suggested I think of my dark mood as a cloud that I could push away," Peri relates. "She told me that whenever I felt a bad spell coming on to close my eyes and picture myself blowing at that cloud until it disappeared. At first I resisted, but once I gave it a chance, I found it helped a lot."

Although it is possible to conduct your own guided imagery sessions, it's best to have a trained professional, preferably someone who has experience with treating people with depression, develop a program for you and guide you through the steps until they become familiar. Talk to your therapist if the idea interests you.

Meditation: Like biofeedback and guided imagery, meditation is a mental exercise that affects body processes. Meditation is performed for a whole host of reasons—religious, spiritual, and physical. When it comes to stress reduction, the purpose of meditation is to gain control over your thoughts so that you can focus on allowing the stress to flow out of your body. Meditation for relaxation requires no special training, and can be done at any time of the day, and in any comfortable space. All it takes is about fifteen minutes of uninterrupted quiet.

Meditation is effective in both reducing general stress and in helping to relax a body and mind made tense by anxiety or worry. When you meditate, you quiet your nervous system, thereby reducing your heart rate and state of muscle contraction. Meditation can help you psychologically by allowing you to focus on the cause of your stress and to find ways to change the way you respond to the challenges you face. Researchers have found when you meditate on a regular basis, you come away with more positive feelings after a stressful encounter, sleep better, and tackle your challenges with more confidence.

"For me, meditation brought a sense of balance to my life," Gail says. "When I meditate, I close my eyes and imagine a round, soft pink ball in the pit of my stomach. This is my center. I see it there, weighing me down in a positive way, keeping me rooted in the here and now, but ready to move and sway and roll with whatever comes up. It really helps."

The Relaxation Response: One easy way to relax is to learn what is known as "the relaxation response." Developed in the 1970s by Herbert Benson, M.D., to counteract the fight or flight response during times of stress, the relaxation response works to bring the body back into balance quickly and efficiently. Here's a deep breathing exercise that may help you trigger this relaxation response whenever you begin to feel overstressed:

1. Sit on the floor in a comfortable position with your back straight and your head erect.

2. Close your eyes and concentrate only on your breath-

ing. Leave behind the worries of the day and think only of this moment in time. Feel your breath as it flows into your mouth and nose and down into your lungs.

3. As you breathe in, picture your body filling with energy, light, and air. Feel your chest and your upper back open up as air enters the area. The inhalation should take about five seconds.

4. When your lungs feel comfortably full, stop the movement and the intake of air. Then exhale in a controlled, smooth continuous movement, with the air streaming steadily out of your nostrils.

5. Repeat the inhalation-exhalations about four times a minute, resting about two or three seconds between breaths, until you feel better.

6. If you like, add a self-affirmation to your relaxation session by saying to yourself, "I am in control. I am relaxed. I can manage my life" or another positive thought every time you exhale.

Practice this relaxation technique as soon as you begin to feel overwhelmed by stress. You might find it especially helpful at work, when trying to cope with the demands of your job might otherwise overwhelm and paralyze you.

These simple relaxation methods, and others, can help you both cope with day-to-day stress-related challenges as well as help you imagine a path to longer-term peace and stability.

COPING WITH DEPRESSION IN THE WORKPLACE

"Work has been a nightmare for me," Marjorie admits. "Part of the stress that triggered my depression in the first place was the pressure I felt to retire. I'm sixty-six and work in an insurance office. It doesn't have an official retirement policy, but I just know they're looking for any reason to fire me and move up one of the younger women. I'm so afraid that my depression would be just the excuse they needed."

Unfortunately, Marjorie is right to be concerned. Despite the fact that we're all living longer and with more vitality than ever before, ageism remains a problem in the workplace and in society. In Marjorie's case, the problem is complicated by the fact that she is struggling with a rather severe depression, a mental illness not always understood or accepted as a genuine medical condition requiring special treatment.

If you're worried about how you should deal with your depression at work, keep in mind that mental illness is covered by the Americans with Disabilities Act of 1990. This act requires employers to make a "reasonable accommodation" for disabled employees. In the case of depression, that might mean giving you a few months to adjust to medication and altering your schedule to minimize long hours or stressful time crunches. Your boss might allow you extra time off for therapist appointments or even a short leave of absence for more intensive treatment. Of course, if you ask for special accommodations, you obviously have to tell your boss about your condition, something that you may find difficult to do.

"I finally had to tell my boss what was going on," Marjorie recounts. "I was surprised at his reaction. He told me he understood because his brother had a problem with depression, and that he'd help as much as he could. He did warn me, though, that there were changes coming in the office—more computers, different accounting systems—that I'd need to keep up with. I'm not sure what I'm going to do, but I do feel better that he'll give me a little more time to adjust."

Marjorie was lucky. Others in her position might well

have been fired, not just because they were depressed but because they could not fulfill their job responsibilities. It's impossible to advise you about what to do at your job without knowing your specific situation. However, there are some general suggestions you might want to consider to make your life at work a little more manageable until you've got your symptoms under control:

▼ *Find support.* Telling your boss and colleagues about your depression may or may not be wise, but if at all possible, you should tell at least one person at work about your condition. Preferably, that person should be someone organized and willing to help you better manage your time and energy. He or she can pick up the slack when you're feeling low, help you stay focused, remind you of important meetings or upcoming projects, and help keep you motivated.

▼ *Take advantage of your "up" times.* If you have flexibility in setting your work schedule, plan to tackle especially creative or intellectually demanding tasks during times of the day when you're apt to feel more energized and focused.

"I've always felt better in the mornings," Jordan admits, "so I try to get up in the morning and go straight into the office to write. I save errands and research for the afternoons. If I don't get them done, it's no big deal. The important thing is getting the words onto paper, at least at this point."

FACING THE FUTURE WITH OPTIMISM

▼ Marilyn, now twenty, plans to return to school in the fall. She's sleeping better now, and that alone has helped return a sense of balance and control to her. She works with a therapist twice a week to sort through her feelings about herself, her parents, and the future. "I'm learning how much more there is to me than what I think others see," Marilyn admits. "It's not that what my friends and family think of me isn't important, but I'm not so worried now about trying to fit anyone's image—including my own—of what my life is supposed to be like. That's really helped to take the pressure off. I still need to learn to pace myself better, and not take on too much, but I'm getting there."

▼ "I can't believe how much of a difference the medication has made in calming me down and getting me focused," Gail recounts. "It hasn't made being a mother any easier, but I do feel so much less overwhelmed by it all. My husband and I are seeing a marriage therapist, not because we have any real deep problems, but just to learn how to talk to each other more openly and directly, how to ask each other for help in more constructive ways. What I want to do now is learn to structure my days a little bit better so that I have some time to develop some interests of my own. I love my baby—he's the best—but I have to work at not feeling so isolated from the 'world of the grown-ups'!"

▼ Beth still can't quite shake her feelings of hopelessness and despair. "I do feel better, and both my new therapist and the medication are helping I guess," she shrugs. "But something is still missing. Something that's been missing all my life. I'm seeing an analyst now and we're looking at my childhood a little more intensely. It makes me feel uncomfortable in some ways, but maybe, finally, we'll figure out what's been dragging me down all these years. Then I'll be able to open up with my kids again, and maybe even try to—oh boy—start dating again!"

▼ "I just celebrated my eighty-third birthday," Gloria says with a smile, "and I'm not giving up now. I did find my husband and me a pretty nifty new place to live, with a golf course nearby for him and a library for me to work in. I've decided to look over my diaries—I've always kept one— and see if I might turn them into some kind of memoir. Not to publish or anything, just for me. To look back at the times of my life and put them into some kind of perspective. I'm excited about it."

Four women, all in different stages of life, all from different socioeconomic and psychosocial backrounds, all with very distinct personalities. What they had in common at the beginning of the book was the depression with which they all suffered. Today, they share the gratifying experience of coming through the darkness to look at their challenges—past, present, and future—with new energy, commitment, and confidence. By no means have they been "cured," but they have learned to accept themselves with more grace, to recognize their strengths, and to cope with the stresses and demands of daily life in more positive ways.

If you're not careful, depression can, and often does, become a chronic condition. Beth, for instance, has suffered off and on from depression all her life. One reason it has become a recurring problem for her is that she never adequately treated it, nor did she quickly get help whenever she noticed symptoms returning.

Because depression is a biochemical disease, often with a built-in genetic component, you may always be vulnerable to depression. You should never blame yourself for not being strong enough to "fight it off" or feel responsible for any relapse you might suffer down the road. There are, however, some ways to minimize your risks of relapse. They include:

▼ *Finding the right treatment.* You may not find the right therapist on the first try, nor will the first medication you try necessarily be the one to lift your spirits and readjust your biochemistry. Although energy and drive may be just what you lack at this time, it's vital that you keep at it until you find what works for you. Only with treatment will you reduce your risks of both sinking deeper into depression or relapsing in just a few months time.

▼ *Taking your medication as prescribed.* If you and your therapist decide you would benefit from an antidepressant or other medication, follow directions with care. Take the medication in the doses prescribed and for as long as your doctor recommends. Your instinct may be to stop taking the medication as soon as you feel better, but this would be a mistake. Studies have shown that patients are more likely to relapse if they stop taking medicine too soon. You'll probably want to take your medication for about six months to a year, but discuss the matter with your doctor.

▼ *Contacting your doctor immediately if you start to feel depressed again.* Watch for signs that depression may be returning. Are you starting to withdraw from your normal activities? Do you tire more easily than normal? Has your appetite changed? Are you more easily frustrated? Have you caught yourself crying at odd or inappropriate times? As soon as you feel you might be suffering a relapse, get into treatment. By doing so you may be able to prevent another full-blown depressive episode from taking hold.

▼ *Taking good care of your general health.* Remember, mind and body are one and the same. Your brain and your spirit need the nutrients found in a good diet, the energy derived from healthy exercise, and the rejuvenation that comes with restful sleep and relaxation.

▼ *Reaching out to others.* You are not alone. If there's any message we hope you've received from this book loud and clear, it's that one. Not only are there people you know and love who can help you, but literally millions of men and women who've traveled the very same dark road you've been on. Reach out to them, ask them for advice, learn from their experiences—and share your own with them.

In the next section, you'll find a list of organizations that can provide you with further information about depression and other mental disorders. These groups can refer you to qualified therapists and support groups in your area, as well as send you pamphlets about the symptoms of depression, the medication and other therapy available to treat it, and the research into its causes and treatment now being conducted in laboratories around the world.

As you begin to come to terms with the effects that depression has had on your life—both positive and negative, and as your symptoms slowly but surely dissipate, you will no doubt find your life becoming more balanced, more structured, and more satisfying.

▼

APPENDIX 1

Resources

Depression is a serious and often isolating illness. It's important for you to keep in mind that you are not alone, and that there is plenty of help out there for you. The associations listed below offer information, most of it free, about every aspect of depression and other mental illnesses. If you want to know more about depression, feel free to make use of these resources to help educate yourself and your family.

Organizations

American Anorexia/Bulimia Association, Inc.
165 West 46th Street, Suite 1108
New York, NY 19936
(212) 575-6200
http://www.aabainc.org

Information on eating disorders and referrals to clinics, therapists, hospital programs, and support groups can be obtained by writing or calling this association.

American Psychiatric Association
1400 K Street, NW
Washington, DC 20005
(202) 682-6000
http://www.psych.org

American Psychological Association
750 First Street, NE
Washington, DC 20002-4242
(202) 374-2721
http://www.apa.org

Anorexia Nervosa and Related Eating Disorders
P.O. Box 5102
Eugene, OR 97405
(503) 344 -1144

Anxiety Disorders Association of America
11900 Parklawn Drive, Suite 100
Rockville, MD 20852
(301) 231-9350
http://www.adaa.org

Center for the Study of Anorexia and Bulimia
1 West 91st Street
New York, New York 10024
(212) 595-3449
http://www.4women.org

Depression Awareness, Recognition, and Treatment (D/ART)
Program Department GL
5600 Fishers Lane, Room 10-85

Rockville, MD 20857
(800) 421-4211

D/ART is a federally funded project created by the National Institute of Health providing free brochures and booklets about all aspects of depression.

National Alliance for the Mentally Ill (NAMI)
200 North Glebe Road, Suite 1015
Arlington, VA 22203-3754
(800) 950-6264
http://www.nami.org

The umbrella group for more than one thousand support and advocacy groups, NAMI provides free information on psychiatric illnesses, medicines, and financial concerns related to mental health care. It offers a special brochure about depression in professional women and African Americans.

National Association of Anorexia Nervosa and Associated Disorders
Box 7
Highland Park, IL 60035
(847) 831-3438
http://www.anad.org

This organization operates a phone line from 9 A.M. to 5 P.M. providing free information, telephone counseling, and nationwide referrals to therapists, support groups, and physicians who specialize in eating disorders.

National Depressive and Manic Depressive Association
730 North Franklin, Suite 501
Chicago, IL 60610-3526
(800) 82-NDMDA
http://www.ndmda.org

This organization offers free brochures about depression and bipolar disorders, as well as information about support groups. Membership in NDMDA ($20 per year) entitles you to a quarterly newsletter.

National Foundation for Depressive Illness
P.O. Box 2257
New York, NY 10116
(212) 268-4260
http://www.depression.org

The National Foundation for Depressive Illness offers referrals to specialists in mood disorders as well as an extensive bibliography of books about depression and bipolar disorder.

National Institute of Mental Health
Public Inquiries
6001 Executive Boulevard, Room 8184, MSC 9663
Bethesda, MD 20892-9663
(301) 443-4513
http://www.nimh.nih.gov

National Mental Health Association (NMHA)
National Mental Health Information Center
1021 Prince Street
Alexandria, VA 23314-2971
(800) 969-6642

National Foundation for Depressive Illness, Inc.
P.O. Box 2257
New York, NY 20116-2257
(800) 248-4344

Obsessive Compulsive Foundation
337 Notch Hill Road
North Branford, CT 06471
(203) 315-2190
http://www.ocfoundation.org

▼

APPENDIX II

Further Reading

Reading about the experiences of therapists, researchers, and, above all, other people who suffer with depression can be both comforting and illuminating. Go to your local library or bookstore and see if any of the titles listed below may help you.

Barlow, David H. *Anxiety and Its Disorders.* New York: Guilford, 1988.

Beck, Aaron T. *Love Is Never Enough.* New York: Harper & Row, 1988.

Berger, Diane and Lisa. *We Heard the Angels of Madness: One Family's Struggle with Manic Depression.* New York: William Morrow, 1991.

Bloomfield, Harold H., M.D., and McWilliams, Peter. *How to Heal Depression.* Los Angeles: Prelude Press, 1994.

Braiker, Harriet. *Getting Up When You're Feeling Down: A Woman's Guide to Overcoming and Preventing Depression.* New York: G.P. Putnam's Sons, 1988.

Chan, Connie S. *If It Runs in Your Family: Depression.* New York: Bantam Books, 1993.

Cronkite, Kathy. *On the Edge of Darkness: Conversations about Conquering Depression.* New York: Doubleday, 1994.

DePaulo J. Raymond, Jr., and Keith Russell Ablow. *How to Cope with Depression: A Complete Guide for You and Your Family.* New York: McGraw-Hill, 1989.

Dowling, Colette. *You Mean I Don't Have to Feel This Way?* New York: Scribner's, 1991.

Dukakis, Kitty. *Now You Know.* New York: Simon & Schuster, 1990.

Duke, Patty, and Gloria Hochman. *A Brilliant Madness: Living with Manic-Depressive Illness.* New York: Bantam Books, 1992.

Engler, Jack, and Daniel Goldman. *The Consumers Guide to Psychotherapy.* New York: Fireside, 1992.

Fieve, Ronald R. *Prozac: Questions and Answers for Patients, Family, and Physicians.* New York: Avon, 1994.

Goldberg, Ivan K., M.D. *Questions and Answers about Depression and Its Treatment: A Consultation with a Leading Psychiatrist.* Philadelphia: The Charles Press, 1993.

Goodwin, F.K., and Jamison, K.R. *Manic-Depressive Illness.* New York: Oxford University Press, 1990.

Hirschfeld, Robert. *When the Blues Won't Go Away.* New York: Macmillan, 1991.

Ingersoll, Barbara D., Ph.D., and Goldstein, Sam, Ph.D. *Lonely, Sad, and Angry: A Parent's Guide to Depression in Children and Adolescents.* New York: Doubleday, 1995.

Jamison, Kay Redfield. *An Unquiet Mind: A Memoir of Moods and Madness.* New York: Knopf, 1995.

Klein, Donald F., and Paul H. Wender. *Understanding Depression.* New York: Oxford University Press, 1993.

Klerman, G.L., M.M. Weissman, B. J. Rounsaville, and E.S. Chevron. *Interpersonal Psychotherapy of Depression.* New York: Basic Books, 1984.

Kramer, Peter D. *Listening to Prozac*. New York: Viking, 1993.

McGrath, Ellen, et al., ed. *Women and Depression*. Washington, DC: American Psychological Association, 1990.

Millett, Kate. *The Loony Bin Trip*. New York: Simon & Schuster, 1990.

Oster, Gerald D., Ph.D., and Montgomery, Sarah S., M.S.W. *Helping Your Depressed Teenager: A Guide for Parents and Caregivers*. New York: John Wiley & Sons, 1995.

Papolos, Demitri F., and Janice Papolos. *Overcoming Depression*. New York: HarperCollins, 1997.

Rosenthal, Norman E. *Winter Blues*. New York: Guilford Press, 1993.

Salmans, Sandra. *Depression: Questions You Have . . . Answers You Need*. Allentown, PA: People's Medical Society, 1995.

Sheehy, Gail. *Passages*. New York: E.P. Dutton, 1976.

Sheehy, Gail. *New Passages*. New York: Random House, 1995.

Styron, William. *Darkness Visible: A Memoir of Madness*. New York: Random House, 1990.

Thompson, Tracy. *The Beast: A Reckoning with Depression*. New York: G.P. Putnam's Sons, 1995.

Weissman, M.M. *Mastering Depression: A Patient's Guide to Interpersonal Psychotherapy*. Albany, NY: Graywind Publications, Inc., 1995.

Wurtzel, Elizabeth. *Prozac Nation: Young and Depressed in America*. New York: Houghton Mifflin, 1994.

▼
GLOSSARY

Acetylcholine: A *neurotransmitter* that helps to regulate memory. It is also one of the principal neurotransmitters involved in bodily functions that are automatic, such as sweating and heart rate.

Addiction: A pattern of behavior based on a great physical and/or psychological need for a substance or activity. Addiction is characterized by compulsion, loss of control, and continued repetition of a behavior no matter the consequences.

Agoraphobia: Mental disturbance involving fear of open, crowded, or public spaces as well as the fear of leaving a familiar place or being in a place where escape may be difficult or help unavailable.

Alcoholism: Chronic and extreme physical dependence on alcohol characterized by tolerance to its effects and withdrawal symptoms when consumption is reduced or stopped. This disease involves complex cultural, social, and physical factors.

Amenorrhea: Absence of monthly menstruation often caused by the malfunction of the *hypothalamus, pituitary gland,* ovary, or uterus. Stress and anxiety are among the causes of amenorrhea.

Anhedonia: The inability to experience pleasure and the loss of interest in activities that once offered pleasure. A common symptom of *depression.*

Anorexia nervosa: A chronic, sometimes fatal *eating disorder* involving a loss of appetite or inability to eat that results in malnutrition, severe weight loss, and medical complications. Anorexia is frequently associated with depression.

Antidepressants: Any of a number of drugs used to treat and relieve depression, including *selective serotonin reuptake inhibitors, tricyclic antidepressants,* and *monoamine oxidase inhibitors.*

Antipsychotics: Any of a number of drugs used to treat the symptoms of *psychosis,* including hallucinations and delusions.

Anxiety: Uneasiness, worry, uncertainty, and fear that comes with thinking about an anticipated danger. Anxiety may be a normal reaction to a real threat or occur when no danger exists.

Anxiety disorders: Any of several psychological disorders characterized by inappropriate and excessive physical and emotional symptoms of *anxiety,* such as restlessness, rapid heartbeat and respiration, and fear. *Agoraphobia, obsessive-compulsive disorder, posttraumatic stress disorder,* and *generalized anxiety disorder* are the most common anxiety disorders. Anxiety disorders are frequently associated with depression.

Attention deficit/hyperactivity disorder: A mental disorder characterized by limited attention span, restlessness, distractibility, hyperactivity, and impulsiveness.

Atypical depression: A form of *major depression* involving symptoms that include increased appetite, weight gain, and sleeping more than usual.

Behavioral modification: A type of *psychotherapy* that attempts to change behavior by rewarding a desired behavior and punishing unwanted behavior; substituting a new response to a given stimulus.

Benzodiazepines: Medications used to treat *anxiety disorders*, including Valium and Librium. At least one benzodiazapine, Xanax, has also shown to be effective in treating depression.

Binge eating: An *eating disorder* characterized by uncontrollable eating of a large amount of food in a relatively short amount of time.

Bipolar disorder: A *mood disorder* characterized by recurrent, alternating episodes of *depression* and *mania*. Formerly called manic depression. Persons who have experienced only manic episodes are also referred to as having a bipolar disorder.

Bulimia nervosa: An *eating disorder* involving episodes of *binge eating* followed by vomiting or purging with diuretics and laxatives. Excessive exercising and fasting may also be involved. Bulimia is often associated with depression.

Catecholamines: A group of structurally related *neurotransmitters* including *serotonin, norepinephrine,* and *dopamine,* thought to be involved in the pathology of depression and other emotional disorders.

Chronobiology: The study of internal body rhythms in order to map hormonal, nerve, and immune-system cyclical functions. Some scientists believe that a disruption of normal body rhythms lies at the heart of depression.

Cognitive therapy: A therapeutic approach that considers depression to be result of pessimistic ways of thinking and distorted attitudes about oneself and one's life. The patient is able to relieve depression by learning new ways to think about her situation through role playing, discussion, and assigned tasks.

Cortisol: A *hormone* produced by the body's adrenal glands, which are located above the kidneys. Cortisol is secreted in large amounts during times of stress and also on a cyclical basis according to internal sleep-wake rhythms.

Cushing's disease: A disease in which the adrenal glands are overstimulated and thus produce an overabundance of the hormone *cortisol.* Symptoms of depression and mania may accompany the moonlike facial appearance, unusual fat deposits, and high blood pressure usually seen in this condition.

Delusion: A false belief held persistently despite abundant and clear evidence to the contrary.

Dementia: A cognitive disorder characterized by impaired memory, judgment, language, thinking, and perceptions.

Dopamine: One of the *catecholamine* neurotransmitters that may play a role in depression.

Dual diagnosis: The concurrent occurrence of a psychiatric disorder and a substance disorder in the same individual at the time of diagnosis.

Dysthymia: A chronic depressive state that lasts at least two years with symptoms more mild (but longer lasting) than major depression. Symptoms include feelings of inadequacy, hopelessness, low energy, and an inability to enjoy pleasurable activities.

Electroconvulsive therapy (ECT): The application of electric current to the brain through electrodes attached to the scalp. This electricity induces a convulsive seizure that often helps alleviate depression.

Endocrine system: The network of glands and tissues that produce *hormones* and secrete them into the blood for transport to target organs. Disorders of the endocrine system often cause depressive symptoms.

Endorphins: Chemicals that help to elevate mood and alleviate pain. Low levels of endorphins are related to depression.

Epinephrine: Also called adrenaline, a substance produced by the adrenal gland, often in response to stress. It is responsible for many of the physical manifestations of fear and anxiety.

Estrogen: The sex hormone that plays a major role in the development and maintenance of female secondary sex characteristics.

Family therapy: Therapy that focuses on understanding and/or improving marital partnerships and family relationships as a way to treat an individual's or family's emotional or psychological problems.

Generalized anxiety disorder: An anxiety disorder characterized by unrealistic and excessive apprehension about life circumstances that lasts for more than six months and interferes with normal functioning.

Hormones: Substances secreted by the *endocrine system* that have a specific effect on other organs and processes. Hormones are often referred to as "chemical messengers," and they influence such diverse activities as growth, sexual development, metabolism, and sleep cycles.

Huntington's disease: An inherited and often fatal disease that causes affected individuals to lose their intellectual abilities and become unable to control their movements. Symptoms of depression and/or manic depression often appear early in the course of this condition.

Insomnia: A chronic inability to sleep, or to remain asleep, at night. A variety of factors cause insomnia, including diet and exercise habits, emotional stress, and hormonal imbalances.

Learned helplessness: The passive acceptance of painful or disturbing stimuli after a period during which escape from the stimuli has been blocked. Learned helplessness has been proposed as a potential trigger for depression.

Lithium carbonate: A naturally occurring mineral salt used to treat manic and depressive episodes and bipolar disorder.

L-tryptophan: The major building block of the neurotransmitter *serotonin.*

Mania: The high phase of *bipolar disorder.* Symptoms may include excessive elation, inflated self-esteem, hyperactivity, and rapid and confused speaking and thinking patterns.

Manic-depression: see *bipolar disorder.*

Marital therapy: Therapy intended to improve relationships between married partners.

Monoamine oxidase inhibitors (MAOIs): Antidepressant medication that works by inhibiting monoamine oxidase, an enzyme that breaks down norepinephrine, serotonin, dopamine, and other neurotransmitters.

Narcotic: Any drug that is derived from or has a chemical structure similar to that of an opiate and which relieves pain and alters mood. Most narcotics are *addictive.*

Neurons: Nerve cells; the basic units of the nervous system. Neurons are able to conduct impulses and communicate by releasing and receiving *neurotransmitters.*

Neurotransmitters: Chemicals that result in the sending of nerve signals, including *serotonin, dopamine,* and *norepinephrine* among others. Neurotransmitters are released by *neurons.* When an imbalance occurs, emotional and physical symptoms often result.

Norepinephrine: A *catecholamine neurotransmitter* thought to be involved in affective disorders like depression.

Obsessive-compulsive disorder (OCD): An *anxiety disorder* characterized by recurrent obsessions or compulsions that impair the ability to function in daily life or to form significant relationships. Depression often occurs with OCD.

Panic disorder: Recurrent attacks of panic which involve sudden, unprovoked intense fear or discomfort, usually lasting several minutes. Physical symptoms such as rapid heartbeat, dizziness, nausea, shortness of breath, and feeling as if one is losing control.

Phobia: An unreasonable fear surrounding a specific object, activity, or situation. Phobias are frequently associated with atypical depression.

Phototherapy: Treatment for depression in which the patient is exposed to bright lights for several hours each day. Phototherapy is particularly useful for sufferers of *Seasonal Affective Disorder (SAD)*.

Postpartum depression: A severe and long-lasting depression following childbirth.

Posttraumatic stress disorder (PTSD): An *anxiety disorder* occurring after exposure to extreme mental or physical stress—usually involving death, threatened death, or serious injury—and characterized by symptoms that persist for one month or more. Symptoms include reexperiencing the event, avoidance of stimuli related to it, and, frequently, an associated depression.

Premenstrual dysphoric disorder: An uncommon type of depression related to *premenstrual syndrome* that occurs in the last week of the menstrual cycle.

Premenstrual syndrome: A common condition characterized by physical discomfort and psychological distress that occurs prior to the onset of a woman's menstrual period.

Psychiatrist: A licensed medical doctor who specializes in the diagnosis and treatment of mental and emotional disorders.

Psychoanalysis: A form of therapy originally developed by Sigmund Freud that seeks to identify repressed issues and emotional conflicts from childhood. Techniques involve free association and dream interpretation. The process usually involves frequent sessions—often one hour every day—over a long period of time.

Psychologist: A person with a doctoral degree (Ph.D. or Psy.D.) in psychology that includes training in counseling, psychotherapy, and psychological testing.

Psychoneuroimmunology: The study of how the nervous system and immune system interact in the body.

Psychopathology: The study of the development, symptoms, and nature of mental disorders.

Psychopharmacology: The study of the actions and effects of drugs that work to alter emotions and behavior in people and animals.

Psychotherapy: Treatment for psychiatric disorders involving support, reassurance, and reeducation of the patient.

Psychotropic: A term used to describe the actions of drugs used to treat mental and emotional illness.

Rapid cycling: A condition in *bipolar disorder* in which four or more episodes of mood disturbance (mania, depression, or both) occur within a year or less.

Receptors: Specialized molecules on the surface of *neurons* to which particular *neurotransmitters* attach after their release from another neuron. This binding allows a message to be passed from one neuron to another.

Schizophrenia: A mental disorder characterized by psychotic symptoms such as delusions and hallucinations. The onset is generally between late adolescence and the mid-thirties.

Seasonal affective disorder (SAD): A type of depression that recurs at a particular time of year, usually during the fall and winter months when daylight hours are shortest.

Selective serotonin reuptake inhibitor (SSRI): A type of antidepressant that works to prevent the *reuptake* of the neurotransmitter *serotonin*. This allows messages about emotion and behavior to be sent and received more efficiently.

Self-esteem: A sense of self-worth and of valuing oneself as a person.

Serotonin: A *neurotransmitter* found in the brain and the body involved in behavior, emotion, and appetite.

Side effect: An unintended drug response that accompanies the intended effect of a particular drug.

Stress: Anything that causes an action or reaction in the body, positive or negative, emotional or physical.

Stressor: Any factor—physical or emotional—that has an effect on the body.

Substance abuse: The compulsive use of a substance such as alcohol or drugs despite the ill effects these substances cause to one's emotional, social, and physical well-being.

Suicide: The taking of one's life.

Synapse: The gap between the nerve endings of two *neurons*. For a message to pass across the synapse, it needs help from a *neurotransmitter*.

Thyroid gland: An *endocrine gland* located in the neck.

Tricyclic antidepressants: Any of several antidepressant drugs that have a three-ring chain as part of their chemical structure.

Tyramine: A chemical additive in many foods that can cause a dangerous rise in blood pressure when a drug of the *monoamine oxidase inhibitor* is taken.

Unipolar depression: A mood disorder in which only episodes of depression occur, unlike *bipolar disorder,* in which episodes of both *mania* and depression occur.

INDEX

Look for these other titles in the Woman Doctor's Series from Kensington Publishing:

Menopause: A Woman Doctor's Guide
by
Lois Jovanovic, MD with Suzanne LeVert

PMS: A Woman Doctor's Guide
by
Andrea J. Rapkin, MD, FACOG, with Diana Tonnessen

Infertility: A Woman Doctor's Guide
by
Susan Treiser, MD, with Robin K. Levinson

Miscarriage: A Woman Doctor's Guide
by
Lynn Friedman, MD, with Irene Daria

Skin Care: A Woman Doctor's Guide
by
Wilma F. Bergfeld, MD, with Shelagh Ryan Masline

Osteoporosis: A Woman Doctor's Guide
by
Yvonne, R. Sherrer, MD, with Robin K. Levinson

7110